W9-BYY-306

Pot in Pans

Rowman & Littlefield Studies in Food and Gastronomy

General Editor: Ken Albala, Professor of History, University of the Pacific (kalbala@pacific.edu)
Rowman & Littlefield Executive Editor: Suzanne Staszak-Silva (sstaszak-silva@rowman.com)

Food studies is a vibrant and thriving field encompassing not only cooking and eating habits but also issues such as health, sustainability, food safety, and animal rights. Scholars in disciplines as diverse as history, anthropology, sociology, literature, and the arts focus on food. The mission of **Rowman & Littlefield Studies in Food and Gastronomy** is to publish the best in food scholarship, harnessing the energy, ideas, and creativity of a wide array of food writers today. This broad line of food-related titles will range from food history, interdisciplinary food studies monographs, general interest series, and popular trade titles to textbooks for students and budding chefs, scholarly cookbooks, and reference works.

Appetites and Aspirations in Vietnam: Food and Drink in the Long Nineteenth Century, by Erica J. Peters
Three World Cuisines: Italian, Mexican, Chinese, by Ken Albala
Food and Social Media: You Are What You Tweet, by Signe Rousseau
Food and the Novel in Nineteenth-Century America, by Mark McWilliams
Man Bites Dog: Hot Dog Culture in America, by Bruce Kraig and Patty Carroll
A Year in Food and Beer: Recipes and Beer Pairings for Every Season, by Emily Baime and Darin Michaels
Celebraciones Mexicanas: History, Traditions, and Recipes, by Andrea Lawson Gray and Adriana Almazán Lahl
The Food Section: Newspaper Women and the Culinary Community, by Kimberly Wilmot Voss
Small Batch: Pickles, Cheese, Chocolate, Spirits, and the Return of Artisanal Foods, by Suzanne Cope
Food History Almanac: Over 1,300 Years of World Culinary History, Culture, and Social Influence, by Janet Clarkson
Cooking and Eating in Renaissance Italy: From Kitchen to Table, by Katherine A. McIver
Eating Together: Food, Space, and Identity in Malaysia and Singapore, by Jean Duruz and Gaik Cheng Khoo
Nazi Hunger Politics: A History of Food in the Third Reich, by Gesine Gerhard
The Carrot Purple and Other Curious Stories of the Food We Eat, by Joel S. Denker
Food in the Gilded Age: What Ordinary Americans Ate, by Robert Dirks
Urban Foodways and Communication: Ethnographic Studies in Intangible Cultural Food Heritages around the World, by Casey Man Kong Lum and Marc de Ferrière le Vayer
Food, Health, and Culture in Latino Los Angeles, by Sarah Portnoy
Food Cults: How Fads, Dogma, and Doctrine Influence Diet, by Kima Cargill
Prison Food in America, by Erika Camplin
K'Oben: 3,000 Years of the Maya Hearth, by Amber M. O'Connor and Eugene N. Anderson
As Long as We Both Shall Eat: A History of Wedding Food and Feasts, by Claire Stewart
American Home Cooking: A Popular History, by Tim Miller
A Taste of Broadway: Food in Musical Theater, by Jennifer Packard
Pigs, Pork, and Heartland Hogs: From Wild Boar to Baconfest, by Cynthia Clampitt
Sauces Reconsidered: Après Escoffier, by Gary Allen
Pot in Pans: A History of Eating Cannabis, Robyn Griggs Lawrence

Pot in Pans

A History of Eating Cannabis

Robyn Griggs Lawrence

Foreword by Chris Kilham

ROWMAN & LITTLEFIELD
Lanham • Boulder • New York • London

Published by Rowman & Littlefield
An imprint of The Rowman & Littlefield Publishing Group, Inc.
4501 Forbes Boulevard, Suite 200, Lanham, Maryland 20706
www.rowman.com

6 Tinworth Street, London SE11 5AL, United Kingdom

British Library Cataloguing in Publication Information Available

Library of Congress Cataloging-in-Publication Data
Names: Lawrence, Robyn Griggs, author.
Title: Pot in pans : a history of eating cannabis / Robyn Griggs Lawrence.
Description: Lanham : Rowman & Littlefield, an imprint of The Rowman & Littlefield Publishing Group, Inc., [2019] | Series: Rowman & Littlefield studies in food and gastronomy | Includes bibliographical references and index.
Identifiers: LCCN 2018051090 (print) | LCCN 2018051496 (ebook) | ISBN 9781538106983 (electronic) | ISBN 9781538106976 (cloth : alk. paper)
Subjects: LCSH: Cooking (Marijuana) | Snack foods. | Desserts. | LCGFT: Cookbooks.
Classification: LCC TX819.M25 (ebook) | LCC TX819.M25 L38 2019 (print) | DDC 641.6/379—dc23
LC record available at https://lccn.loc.gov/2018051090

∞™ The paper used in this publication meets the minimum requirements of American National Standard for Information Sciences—Permanence of Paper for Printed Library Materials, ANSI/NISO Z39.48-1992.

Printed in the United States of America

Contents

Foreword

Robyn Griggs Lawrence can't seem to get out of the kitchen, and that is indeed wonderful news for readers. The author of the delightful *The Cannabis Kitchen Cookbook* is still in the kitchen, though apparently with a huge stack of books, articles, obscure references, delightful stories, outlandish events, funny scenes, and hard-to-find facts scattered all about. If information and history were spices, *Pot in Pans* is a fabulously well-seasoned recipe.

Instead of the fragrance of dishes cooking on the stove, Robyn's writing does the tantalizing, hooking your senses until your appetite, stoked by the delicious tale she weaves, moves you to sit down, get comfortable, and read deeply. I can imagine her late at night, combing through references, cross-referring, and getting excited by a new gem, whether it has to do with the hair-splitting definitions that have caused confusion in the world of cannabis or the discovery of a quirky historical character. Simply put, this is a wonderful read, and Robyn evidently had a great time pursuing the long and complex tale of cannabis as a food throughout history. We are the beneficiaries of her long nights and fastidious investigations.

Pot in Pans takes the reader on a merry if bumpy romp through the history of cannabis as food. In the process, Robyn conjures a delectable blend of impressive obscurata (women in Uzbekistan made a traditional cannabis food called *guc-kand*, who knew?) to a wonderful elucidation of key events in the tumultuous history of weed, such as the bullish efforts of America's first drug czar Harry J. Anslinger to malign cannabis and the roots of the Rastafari religion. From Herodotus to Alice B. Toklas to the Beats, Robyn introduces us to the figures who have played influential roles in the trajectory of cannabis throughout culture and shares some of their potent mind-bending recipes. From the grassy pot brownies of Alice B. Toklas to space cakes in the coffee shops of Amsterdam, she wanders the cannabis landscape, making mycelial connections between the Scythians and Harvard, Tantric yogis and the Vietnam War. The story comes together so smoothly and in such an entertaining way, it's easy to fritter the night away going from page one to the end.

The history of cannabis and its consumption as a food is one of intrigue, false narratives, ardent advocates, belligerent opponents, sneaky recipes, jubilant hash eaters, ham-fisted law-enforcement agencies, stoned literati, and a collection of characters that define diversity itself. It is also the tale of a tough plant that has survived not only the last ice age but the slings and arrows of misfortune, misrepresentation, idiocy, deceit, treachery, and a litany of lies heaped high and piled deep. I found myself reading Robyn's account with laughter, rage, and more than a few shakes of my head, following the serpentine curves of this plant's maneuvers through human history.

One theory that many plant aficionados subscribe to is that plants enlist us, that they appeal to us *intentionally*, and that we wind up doing their bidding, which is to spread them far and wide, thereby assuring their dispersion and survival. In my decades of plant investigation in various countries, I have often asked botanists, herbalists, and other plant lovers, "Are you working for the plants, or are the plants working for you?" Thus far, everyone has answered the former. There is this sense that the plants are wise and clever, and that they draw us in to toil on their behalf. Following this line, there is little doubt that Robyn Griggs Lawrence has been wooed by cannabis, lured by its siren song, and touched by its profound capacity to impact society. With its culinary applications as a lead, in *Pot in Pans* she has pried open a treasure chest of fascinating cannabis history, legendary characters, improbable events, and a rich tale that will hook you to the last page.

Chris Kilham

Acknowledgments

Thank you to the many professionals who took the time to share their passion and educate me, including Juan Ayala, Peter Barsoom, Missy Bradley, Ziggy Braun, Dr. Andrew Chadeayne, Jon Cooper, Derek Cumings, Scott Durrah, Vaughn Halyard, Zoe Helene, Wanda James, Chris Kilham (above and beyond, as always!), Elise McDonough, Noel Palmer, Randy Placeres, Dr. Brian Reed, Chris Sayegh, Phil Scarpello, Andrew Schrot, Mindy Segal, and Nancy Whiteman. Many thanks to Suzanne Gerber and Joanna Pruess for spotting this opportunity and passing it along. Thanks to Meryl Davids Landau for coming up with the title. All love to Dennis Crawford and Stacey and Cree Lawrence, and thank you for putting up with me (again!) during the home stretch. And of course, so much gratitude to Ken Albala and Suzanne Staszak-Silva for believing in (and waiting for) this book.

Introduction

> The temporal and spatial diffusion of the plant lies at the intersections of Foucauldian biopolitics, ethnobotany, and political ecology, the moral politics of desire and its control, and world-systems theory, a nexus of relations that plays out at multiple spatial scales ranging from international geopolitics to the rhythms of everyday life. The use of cannabis, and repeated attempts to regulate and curtail it, reflect changing and spatially uneven sets of social norms and practices that reflect the outlooks and strategies both of users and various state and religious bodies that have sought to marginalize it.
>
> —Barney Warf, *High Points: An Historical Geography of Cannabis*

It's already eighty-plus degrees and the air is thick as milk at 10 a.m., as we kick up swarms of biting insects and try to avoid thickets of thorny cat's claws on the rugged trail to Royal's farm. Tucked away on top of a mountain in Orange Hill, where the best cannabis in Jamaica is said to grow, the farm is worth the climb (and the perspiration streaming from every part of me).

Royal's pride is as palpable as the sweet smoke from his spliff as he leads us through a semichaotic patch of knee-high plants growing in old tires, which he promises are "200 percent organically grown," and shows us a shack where branches with sticky, fragrant flowers hang from ropes strung in the rafters to dry and cure. As Royal lets each of us examine the medal he won for "best indica strain" at the Cannabis Cup in Negril the year before, his grandchildren chat and pose for photos with us, and we talk about what a blessing it is that Royal and his family no longer have to worry about the authorities arresting him for his fields of ganja or—worse—eradicating them.

It's December 2017, and two years earlier Jamaica decriminalized adult use of cannabis and legalized medical marijuana, determined as a nation to get its rightful piece of a multibillion-dollar industry built around a plant the island helped make famous around the world. For Jamaican farmers like Royal, and the industry that revolves around their crop, the new laws mark the end of more than a century of brutal oppression and control based on a plant they consider sacred.

A week later, I'm back home in Colorado, wearing a white lab coat, hair tucked into a white paper cap, visiting a laboratory-cum-factory in east Denver where Stillwater makes water-soluble powders from cannabis distillate. Keith Woelfel, a food scientist who spent twenty years at Mars, Inc., before he came to Stillwater to figure out how to make molecules that like to dissolve in fat dissolve in water, is explaining the great lengths to which his team went to create a tasteless, odorless, calorie-free powder that offers consistent dosing and flavor without the hashy, green bitterness the plant can impart.

While Keith shows me his "secret sauce" method of tumbling and misting tea leaves in a big, mechanical barrel to coat them with the water-soluble powder, slow and steady, I chat with brand director Missy Bradley about the challenges of marketing Stillwater's innovative products. The sterile, windowless, fluorescent-lit room couldn't be farther away from or more different than Royal's farm, but the pride in product and exhilaration about the future that I feel here are the same.

Another week later, on January 1, 2018, I'm in San Diego for the first day of legal cannabis sales to adults in California, where analysts are projecting the industry will be worth $7 billion within a few years. Hundreds of people arrive even before Urbn Leaf, "a feel-good drug boutique" in San Diego's Linda Vista neighborhood, opens its doors. They wait for hours to be among the first nonpatients to purchase half-ounces of Bubba Kush and Classic OG, budder and live resin, CBD-infused lavender drops, and Pot Rocks from Urbn Leaf's well-stocked shelves.

The line snakes out the door all day, fed continuously by waves of people from a big, black party bus that loops around to the beaches and back. Throughout the city, thousands of people swarm the new cannabis stores as twenty-some drivers navigate San Diego's freeways to deliver cannabis and cannabis products. There are raffles and live music concerts. San Diego city officials hope to raise millions of dollars in tax revenue.

There's a #legalizedit jubilance here, too—though not for everyone. Many of the small growers and manufacturers who supplied the never-really-regulated medical marijuana industry in California are being pushed out. The big players in agriculture, food, and technology are moving in, fast. Growers in Northern California's Emerald Triangle, the area encompassing Humboldt, Mendocino, and Trinity counties that served as the cannabis basket for much of the United States for decades, are struggling to compete with industrial growers in more central locations, where it's easier to ship the commodity throughout the vast state. For generations of families that have sustained themselves growing cannabis, which thrived in the region's rich terroir with its ample sunshine and nourishing ocean breezes, a way of life is unraveling.

Locally, nationally, and globally, we've reached a pivotal moment in the history of a plant that has been beloved by the masses, reviled by the elite, and shrouded in conflict and secrecy for centuries. Cannabis has been outlawed and demonized since the powers-that-be first realized they could control the commoners by prohibiting a plant that they relied on for food, fiber, medicine, and mind and mood alteration. For the hard-working classes, who often lived in hopeless poverty, cannabis was magical for its ability to act as both stimulant and soporific and its promise of gentle relief from the drudgery and humiliations of daily life—a far cry from the sinister reputation foisted upon it by centuries of propaganda. We are reaching the end of a centuries-long story, born in the Mazandaran mountains in ancient Persia in the twelfth century and used throughout history in racist campaigns to prove that cannabis makes people violent, insane, and uncontrollably horny (*parents, hold onto your white daughters!*). The legend of Hassan-ibn-Sabbah, the Old Man of the Mountain who plied his disciples with splendid food, fine women, and a hashish confection so they would assassinate his enemies—popularized in the West by explorer Marco Polo—would forever associate hashish with assassins and sinister business.

In the 1930s, during his successful drive toward cannabis prohibition, US Federal Bureau of Narcotics chairman Harry J. Anslinger masterfully fomented Americans' racist and increasingly moralistic national mentality with a propaganda blitzkrieg that included a book and motion picture titled *Marihuana: Assassin of Youth*—based upon his discovery of the Old Man of the Mountain legend. In testimony before Congress and in newspaper interviews, Anslinger said that marijuana, a frightening "new" drug used primarily by Mexicans and African Americans, could turn upstanding, middle-class kids into helpless victims and raging monsters. His campaign resulted in cannabis being effectively outlawed through draconian taxes and regulations in the Marihuana Tax Act of 1937.

Down through the ages—through multiple prohibitions on every continent, imposed by sultans, colonialists, and a pope—cannabis had managed to somehow survive, and even thrive. But never had it faced an enemy so formidable or iron-fisted as the United States in the mid-twentieth century. When US Treasury Secretary Andrew W. Mellon appointed Anslinger and tasked him, for whatever reason—and speculation is rampant—to wipe out cannabis, he intended the war to be global. Throughout the rest of the twentieth century and into the twenty-first, the United States used its considerable influence to force cannabis prohibition around the world, leaving people in countries where it had been used and enjoyed for centuries scratching their heads in confusion—and finding ways around the laws.

In Canada in the 1930s, when Royal Mounted Police officers told an elderly woman they had to eradicate the hemp plants she grew to feed her canaries, she chased them away with a broom. In Indonesia, cannabis continued to be a key ingredient in the traditional "happy" soup served at weddings and celebrations, just as it always had. India managed to keep on the right side of the United States while quietly allowing people to drink *bhang*, a traditional holy drink made from cannabis. By the 1970s, the Netherlands had adopted a policy of tolerance toward retailers and users while making cannabis cultivation and production illegal, creating a "back door" problem that no one wanted to replicate.

It was more than clear by the 1970s that the global war on drugs was a failure. Violent cartels were ravaging South and Central America, and heroin, cocaine, and cannabis remained readily available to those who wanted them. In the early and mid-1970s, several countries and US states decriminalized cannabis, but this attitude change was short-lived, squelched by marijuana's association with dirty hippies and the counterculture. The Nixon administration doubled down, sending military helicopters to scorch cannabis farms from Orange Hill to the mountains of Colombia's Cauca region and declaring cannabis a Schedule 1 drug with no medicinal value, alongside heroin and LSD.

For a century now, cannabis has existed in most parts of the world only because humans' love for it is so great that they're willing to sacrifice being persecuted, imprisoned, having their teeth pulled out, and even being put to death for cultivating and nurturing it. The irony of prohibition, of course, is that the lucrative black market made it worth the risk and only drove breeders to develop ever-mightier plants delivering whopping amounts of psychoactive tetrahydrocannabinol, or THC. In the face of adversity, cannabis was no shrinking violet. The plant grew stronger, better, faster, and more potent—unstoppable, no matter how much paraquat the DEA threw at it.

If the history of cannabis proves anything, it is that you can't keep a good plant down. A cabal of global elites is no match for this one, which in its cunning evolved to provide humans with nutrition, fiber, medicine, and, if you believe many ethnobotanists, the ability to make huge mental and spiritual leaps as a species. Had it not been for the latter—all due to the presence of that THC molecule—this would be a boring book about a multifaceted, utilitarian plant that served humans in many different capacities for centuries.

This is not that.

This is a story with many layers, spanning many continents, held together by the thread of an Islamic confection created to inspire a band of twelfth-century *fedayeen*, which was ported throughout the Middle East, Central Asia, and beyond, invoking hilarity and hostility wherever it went. Inspired by this legend, Western intellectuals and literati, and then the masses, discovered and enjoyed cannabis, hashish, and majoun for much of the mid-nineteenth century and into the 1930s, when Anslinger shut that down.

This is the story of how Brion Gysin, an expatriate artist and writer in Tangier, discovered majoun, typed up a recipe, and sent it to Alice B. Toklas, an expat writer in Paris, to include in a cookbook published in New York and London, causing a minor scandal in the mid-twentieth century and leading to a major mix-up in a major motion picture that morphed majoun into the pot brownie, and turned the pot brownie into a Western icon forevermore. It's the story of the rowdy band of artists, rebels, and intellectuals who partook of majoun's charms and an activist who made the pot brownie a symbol of compassion. Down through the ages, the cannabis plant has gathered about it a charismatic and eclectic assortment of protectors and advocates, from the Hindu lord Shiva, who was said to sustain himself for long periods by eating cannabis, to Brownie Mary, whose insistence on baking cannabis-laced brownies as medicine for AIDS patients in San Francisco, despite several arrests, drew huge public sympathy in the 1990s and eased the way for California to legalize medical marijuana in 1996.

And that, really, may have been the beginning of the end of the pot brownie. Several states and countries followed California in approving cannabis for medical use, and in 2012, Colorado and Washington voters took the game-changing step of legalizing all adult use. More states followed, then Uruguay, then Canada. Cannabis-infused edibles grew into a robust and well-regulated industry with no room for crumbly chocolate cakes that had miserable shelf lives and were impossible to imprint with the new THC warning stamp some states began requiring.

In most cases, pot brownies have evolved into shelf-stable, easier-to-dose chocolate bars, one skew in a wildly popular category of cannabis-infused products that no one saw coming in the early 2010s. In addition to a range of chocolate products from gourmet truffles to peanut butter cups, today's cannabis consumers can enjoy infused potato chips, gummies, hard candies, raw cacao butter, soda pop, caramel corn, coffee, tea, cookies, pies, and nuts—all readily available at cannabis stores in legal states. They can buy water-soluble cannabis-infused liquids and powders like Stillwater's to stir into beverages or add to any recipe for immediate gratification. With such a wide range of culinary opportunities and resources literally at their fingertips, only the laziest or most unimaginative eaters are choosing the brownie.

We stand on a precipice. Once criminalized, cannabis is now being rapidly commodified, and there's no putting that genie back in the bottle. Analysts predict cannabis will be a global industry worth \$57 billion by 2027—investment firm Cowen and Company suggests that will reach \$75 billion by 2030—numbers that are respectful enough to prevent cannabis haters from prosecuting companies working within legal state infrastructures. Money talks.

Money's talking. Scotts Miracle-Gro and Monsanto are circling the nascent cannabis industry. Food conglomerates are dipping toes, preparing to jump in when—and everyone now agrees it's a matter of when—federal cannabis prohibition ends in the United States. When this book went to press, bills had been submitted to Congress to legalize both marijuana and its nonpsychoactive "cousin" hemp, caught in Prohibition's crossfire despite its inability to get anyone high. (In fact, theories abound that it was hemp's utility as paper that invoked the wrath of timber baron and newspaper magnate William Randolph Hearst, who put his considerable muscle behind Anslinger's campaign, but that's a story for a different day.)

What happens next? Writing a history book while debate rages over whether we've crossed a historical line in cannabis legalization—and who's on the right side of it—is an unending task. Colorado and California continue to charge ahead toward unfettered cannabis capitalism, to the chagrin of many, while Canada and Uruguay take steps to make the newly legal industry in their countries as staid and boring as possible. Officials in those countries have witnessed the challenges that edibles have presented in Colorado and California—including increases in accidental ingestion by children and overdoses by adults—and they do not take them lightly.

We're seeing, and will continue to see, a renaissance in the cultivation of hemp and the production of hemp food products, which contain only trace amounts of THC. We'll see imminent and widespread acceptance and legalization of cannabidiol (CBD), the other primary cannabinoid in cannabis that provides therapeutic value without psychoactive effects. We will, finally, be able to do the research to understand how and why these molecules work together and with our bodies to provide healing, nutrition, and relief.

Cannabis is now the second most valuable crop in the United States after corn. In 2018, four years after its voters legalized adult use, Oregon held its first-ever cannabis growers' fair to educate people about the state's new legal commodity. That same year, the Specialty Food Association listed cannabis edibles among the top ten food trends in the United States. "In much of the United States, cannabis is no longer inherently edgy," a J. Walter Thompson white paper reported. "If anything, it's moved towards the realms of Instagram gurus and soccer moms."[1]

Chefs, foodies, and nutritionists will continue to play with and perfect this new functional food ingredient, finding creative uses for every part of the plant, as the world's attitude toward cannabis continues to normalize. Shoppers will be able to pick up cured cannabis flowers and concentrates at the market, and diners will be able to sit down in restaurants and enjoy cannabis-infused lentil soup or chia bowls without fear of the law.

This may sound far-fetched, particularly to people who live in places where cannabis remains illegal, where citizens—inordinately, people of color—are rotting in jail because of a plant. For many people of my mother's generation, who were drilled early and often with Anslinger's propaganda about the plant's evils, it may never seem quite right. We have a century of lies and misinformation, based on ignorance and deep racism, to undo.

It will never be okay that (mostly) white men in suits rake in millions of dollars on cannabis and cannabis products while others go to jail over the very same plant. As we celebrate the strides we've made toward liberating cannabis, we must never forget that this progress has been made on the backs of those willing to pay the price before us.

Sitting in Royal's yard under a lush canopy of tree branches and ferns on that muggy December day in Orange Hill, as he cradles his Cannabis Cup medallion in his hand and talks about what a difference the relaxation of Jamaica's ganja laws has made for him and his family, I get a sense of what the new normal will be like. One day, I hope, I'll be able to stop by and have a nice visit with a local farmer like Royal as I pick up 200 percent organically grown cannabis for dinner—no matter where I live.

Bob Marley famously said that cannabis could heal nations. The healing of nations begins with a single household. The time has come for everyone, everywhere, to experience the full joy I found at Royal's.

• 1 •

Cavepeople Ate Cannabis

Like everything else about the cannabis plant, its origins, evolution, and taxonomy are shrouded in mystery and have been the subject of heated debate among botanists, ethnobotanists, and historians since cannabis entered modern taxonomic literature in 1753. Even its name, *Cannabis sativa*, is controversial. Unfortunately, global prohibition has prevented the research necessary to resolve the mysteries surrounding this promiscuous colonizing plant, which, it is generally agreed, evolved somewhere in Asia and was carried to every corner of the globe by humans who valued it for food, fiber, recreational intoxication, and spiritual exploration. For millions of years, wild cannabis has been crossing easily between lineages domesticated by humans to produce viable, resilient offspring as the plant has made its way to every corner of the globe.

Through the years, botanists and historians have made good cases in taxonomic literature that sun-loving *Cannabis sativa* got its start everywhere from Mongolia and southern Siberia on the Central Asian steppes to the Huang He River Valley to the Hindu Kush mountains to South Asia to Afghanistan. There is no agreed-upon answer to this day, though there's general consensus that the plant's angiosperms originated during the early to middle Jurassic period in an arid upland habitat. The earliest purported cannabis angiosperm fossils were found in East Asia, which suggests they originated in Southeast Asia and radiated out from there, most likely carried by humans.[1]

In the wild, cannabis plants produce small seeds that burst open easily and fall to the ground, making them inedible. Early humans in search of nutrition likely began cultivating cannabis so they could harvest those

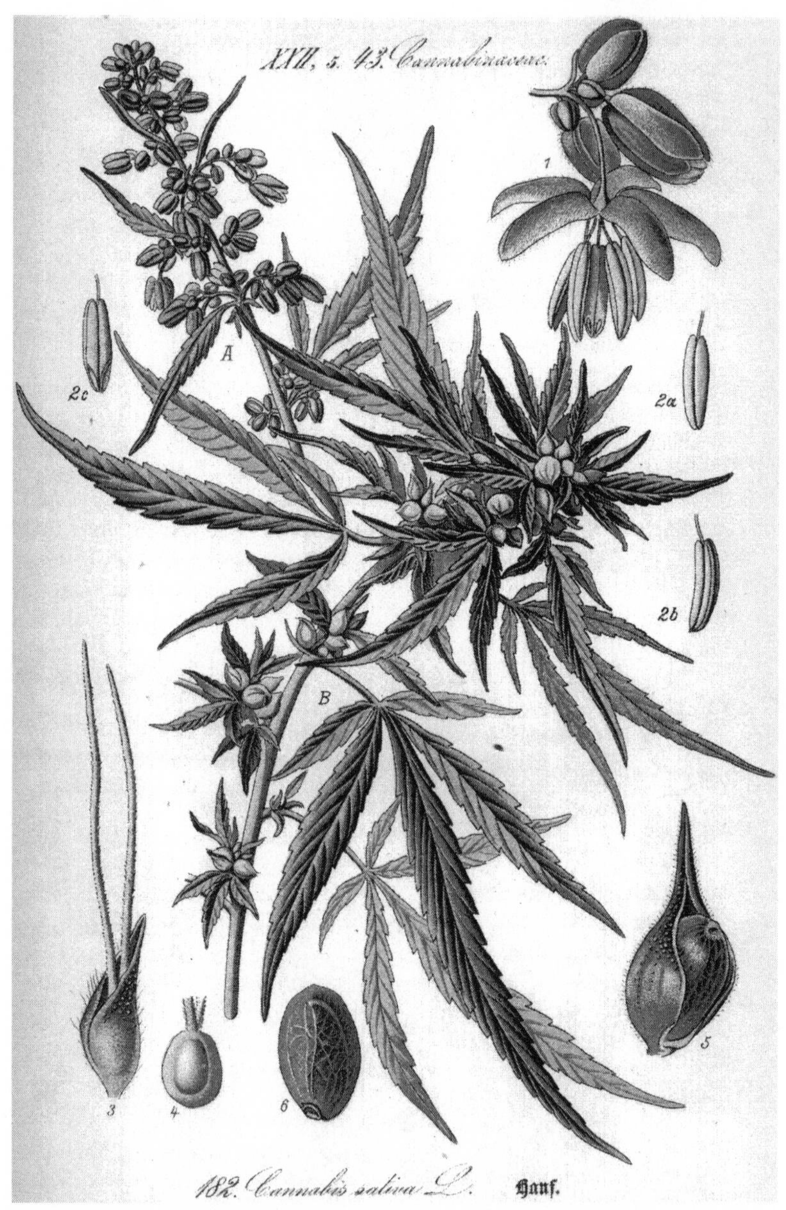

Cannabis sativa. Original book source: Professor Dr. Otto Wilhelm Thomé, *Flora von Deutschland Österreich und der Schweiz* (1885), Gera, Germany. Permission granted to use under GFDL by Kurt Stueber.

seeds beginning in the late Mesolithic period. During Neolithic times, people built communities near freshwater sources and began cultivating crops, including cannabis, which they grew for its edible fruits, fiber, and psychoactive properties, then nomads brought it with them as they traveled from the Black Sea to Mongolia. The Scythians, a tribe of Neolithic migrants, carried hemp seeds to India, China, and Europe, where human communities began selecting and breeding plants to work within their climates and meet their needs for food, fiber, medicine, recreation—or all four—which resulted in the development of a diverse range of strains adapted to live on every continent on the planet.

Exactly when cannabis evolved is another subject of debate, though it's widely believed to be among the first plant life that humans discovered. Botanists John McPartland and Geoffrey Guy of London-based GW Pharmaceuticals presented genetic analysis at the 2010 International Cannabis Research Society's annual meeting suggesting the cannabis plant diverged around 27.8 million years ago from *Humulus*, or hops.[2] Cannabis researcher Robert C. Clarke of the International Hemp Association in Amsterdam and University of Hawaii botanist Mark D. Merlin believe the plant survived the Pleistocene ice ages before it colonized most of Eurasia during the early Holocene warming and then, over millions of years, was transported by humans to nearly every temperate and subtropical region in the world. "Taken as a whole," Clarke and Merlin wrote in *Cannabis: Evolution and Ethnobotany*, "Cannabis presently grows in a wider variety of natural and human-created niches than probably any other plant."[3]

Swedish botanist Carolus Linnaeus, known as the father of modern taxonomy, launched a centuries-long debate about cannabis nomenclature when he introduced a resilient and prolific new species that he had named after the Greek word *kannabis*, meaning "hemp" in the ancient classical vernacular, in his *Species Plantarum* in 1753. (Richard Evans Schultes, considered by many the father of ethnobotany, later used this etymology to back up his theory that cannabis originated in central Asia. *Kannabis* was "presumably a loan word pointing to Finno-Ugrian and Turkish," which were ancient languages of central Asia, Schultes pointed out.[4]) The word *sativa* means "cultivated," and it refers to the hemp plants that people all across Europe grew to harvest for fiber and nutritious seeds during Linnaeus's time. When Linnaeus recorded the plant, he documented one species with five variants, launching a taxonomical argument that is still not officially resolved.

The argument started thirty years after Linnaeus recorded *C. sativa* in the *Species Plantarum*, when French naturalist Jean-Baptiste Lamarck introduced what he described as a second "very distinct" species, *C. indica*, based on plant samples he had been sent from India, in his *Encyclopedie Methodique*. Unlike the tall, lanky *C. sativa* (hemp) that was common in Europe, Lamarck described *C. indica* as smaller and more densely branched, with consistently alternating leaves and a woodier stem that made the plant unsuitable for making fiber. Lamarck wrote that there were two separate species of cannabis, *Chanvre cultive* ("cultivated hemp") and *Chanvre des Indes* ("Indian cannabis"), which he believed was valued more for its psychoactive effects than its fiber potential. "The principal effect of this plant consists of going to the head, disrupting the brain, where it produces a sort of drunkenness that makes one forget one's sorrows, and produces a strong gaiety," Lamarck wrote.[5]

Lamarck was the first to suggest there was a distinction between two separate species of cannabis based on *C. indica*'s psychoactive effects, and botanists argue to this day about whether the narcotic properties of "Indian cannabis" are its primary virtue. "Lamarck suggested as early as 1783 that the content of the intoxicating principal was higher in *C. indica* than in *C. sativa*," Schultes wrote in 1974. "In the intervening 200 years, during which the epithet indica has been used, there has usually been the inference that it is a more strongly intoxicating form of Cannabis. Unfortunately, however, almost no chemical studies have been made in association with taxonomic studies nor on the basis of voucher specimens."[6] In the years to come, as nearly all cannabis research was shut down by the ever-reaching global war on drugs, Lamarck's is yet another theory that researchers have never been able to properly investigate. The debate he launched in 1783 continues to rage.

To complicate matters further, Russian botanist D. E. Janischewsky proposed a third species, *C. ruderalis*, in 1924. Janischewsky believed this weedy species evolved in the wild in the Volga region, western Siberia, and Central Asia and spread rapaciously throughout northern and central Europe and Russia. Janischewsky named it *ruderalis*, from *ruderal*, meaning "growing in a waste area disturbed by humans," because this species thrived on the garbage dumps and compost piles early human settlements left behind when they moved on to new areas.

Clarke and Merlin called *C. ruderalis* "a putative ancestor of the two modern species, *C. sativa* and *C. indica*," and suggest all three species may have evolved from feral *C. indica* plants that escaped from cultivation. Citing plant distribution studies, paleoclimate modeling, archaeological evidence, and the historical record, they propose that *C. sativa* most likely originated in a temperate region of western Eurasia, possibly in the foothills of the Caucasus Mountains, from "a putative hemp ancestor with diminished biosynthetic potential to produce THC," and early *C. indica* populations "diversified as they were introduced by humans to different geographical regions, where they may have further evolved into the three subspecies."[7]

When the United States launched its all-out war on cannabis in the 1930s, and then renewed efforts in the late 1970s and 1980s, it became extremely difficult, if not impossible, for researchers to delve into the mysteries of a plant that was classified as an illegal drug throughout most of the world. As yellow journalists and US government crusaders shifted public perception of cannabis from medicine to menace in the early twentieth century, virtually all taxonomic discussion and complicated scientific efforts stopped, allowing a lot of incorrect nomenclature to become common vernacular. That is starting to change as prohibition begins to crumble, opening up a space for a cannabis research renaissance being led by Israeli scientists.

But when it comes to cannabis nomenclature, things can always get more complicated. In the 1970s, a furious forensic debate erupted during a trial over a narcotics charge based on the defendant's argument that the name *C. sativa*, which was used to denote "cannabis drugs" in most North American legislation, did not include the other two species, *C. ruderalis* and *C. indica*—which meant that, technically, those species were legal. (The defendant, of course, was caught with *C. indica.*) Schultes, as an expert witness for the defense, publicly changed his earlier position that cannabis was a monospecies and argued that there were three species: *C. sativa*, *C. indica*, and *C. afghanica*. His colleagues all over the world were appalled at the venerated scholar's sharp reversal, and some publicly shamed him for taking part in what Canadian botanists Ernest Small and Arthur Cronquist called "the current cause celebre."[8]

In the twenty-first century, forensic science had a new tool, DNA, to work with—and so did cannabis researchers, as relaxing laws and technological advancements allowed scientists to delve more deeply into the plant. Scientific debate reached an entirely new level as pharmaceutical companies with deep pockets, led by GW Pharmaceuticals, got into the game with varying agendas. In 2014, GW Pharmaceuticals' Dr. John McPartland called on the International Cannabinoid Research

Society to create an accurate vernacular nomenclature for cannabis based on his genetic barcode research, which determined that *C. indica* and *C. sativa* are subspecies of one *Cannabis* species.[9]

Game over? This is cannabis; that would be too easy. The debate continued to spiral through scholarly circles and Internet chat rooms. In states where cannabis use was made legal, "indica" and "sativa" took on an entirely different meaning at dispensaries and retail stores, based not on how they grew or evolved but on their effects (indica soporific and sativa energizing). These descriptions, while convenient, actually had nothing to do with the raging species debates within botanical circles and weren't based on science. They were so prolific, however, that the labels became commonly accepted "knowledge" in the industry.

Whether he intended it to or not, Lamarck gave people an easy-to-understand formula for distinguishing between plants with very different functions. In a *Cannabinoids 2014* article titled "That Which We Call *Indica*, by Any Other Name Would Smell as Sweet," Jacob L. Erkelens and Arno Hazekamp explained that Lamarck's purpose in classifying *C. indica* as a separate species was to provide a more generally acceptable description of the cannabis. "Unfortunately, the long-term effects of his publication would turn out to do the exact opposite," they wrote, "and well over two hundred years later we are still left in confusion."[10]

Parts of the Plant

Flower: Egg- or conical-shaped clusters of blooms that grow up to several inches long.
Cola: Cluster of female flowers that can grow up to a foot in length.
Trichome: Tiny hairs with sticky crystal resin glands on leaves, stems, and calyxes.
Calyx: Tear-shaped nodule underneath sugar leaves with high concentrations of trichomes.
Pistil: Tiny, red-orange hair that collects pollen.
Fan Leaf: Large, pointy leaves, mostly devoid of trichomes, removed at harvest.
Sugar Leaf: Small, resin-coated leaves trimmed from flowers during harvest.

A TASTE TEST THAT LED TO RELIGION

During the Stone Age, humans began exploring their surroundings and figuring out how to survive, forming crude communities along freshwater sources and experimenting with eating the plants and animals they encountered. These humans would have had a hard time ignoring the cannabis plant, its pungent flowers dripping with resin, and ethnobotanists believe it was one of the very first plants they explored. The cavepeople tasted cannabis's fresh green leaves, bitter flowers, and nutty seeds. The thick sap coating the flowers, rich with THC, stuck to their fingers. When they licked it off, they discovered the plant's ability to intoxicate. They were the first in a long line of hash eaters to come.

Today we understand that it was the cannabinoids in the sticky resin of those plants that got those early humans high by activating special human receptors that enhance the expression of FOXP2, a gene that facilitates speech and language development. For our ancestors, there was only an understanding that this plant could take their minds to new places and open up untapped avenues of thought. It gave them good ideas. Researchers Geoffrey Guy and John McPartland theorized that as cannabis coevolved alongside humans, it was primarily responsible for what historians call "the great leap,"[11] the time when we began making tools, weapons, and art, and working together in collectives.

Ethnobotanist Richard Evans Schultes's theory is that ingesting those cannabis plants led early humans to invent religion. "Primitive man, trying all sorts of plant materials as food, must have known the ecstatic hallucinatory effects of Hemp, an intoxication introducing him to another-worldly plane leading to religious beliefs," Schultes and Albert Hofmann wrote in *Plants of the Gods* in 1979. "Thus the plant early was viewed as a special gift of the gods, a sacred medium for communion with the spirit world."[12] Though it was seemingly discovered by accident, Robert C. Clarke and Mark D. Merlin wrote that the female cannabis flowers' ability "to exude large amounts of readily apparent and easily collected psychoactive resin" was the plant's "most evolutionary significant trait."[13]

Though valued for its nutritious seeds, cannabis's psychoactive qualities may well have been the magic bond that motivated early humans to begin putting crops in the ground and continue to plant cannabis wherever they went. After observing that early African Pygmies learned to cultivate cannabis because they considered it an important tool for keeping the hunters soothed and amused during the long hours they spent stalking meat and fish, scientist and author Carl Sagan famously suggested it would be "wryly interesting if in human history the cultivation of marijuana led generally to the invention of agriculture, and thereby to civilization." Sagan went on to observe: "The marijuana-intoxicated Pygmy, poised patiently for an hour with his fishing spear aloft, is earnestly burlesqued by the beer-sodden riflemen, protectively camouflaged in red plaid, who, stumbling through the nearby woods, terrorize American suburbs each Thanksgiving."[14]

As hunter-gatherers moved from place to place in search of food, they left behind campsites of rich compost where wild cannabis seeds germinated and flourished. Later, a vast, wandering, Stone Age religio-complex of tribes seeking new lands and new consciousness brought cannabis, which they used as a spiritual tool, as they traveled farther and wider. Cannabis, Schultes wrote, "developed together with man as a multi-purpose economic plant: the source of a fibre, a narcotic, a medicine, an oil, and an edible fruit."

As soon as they could figure out how to do so, humans domesticated cannabis and began breeding it to enhance useful traits such as elongated bast fibers, large seeds with high oil content, and, sometimes, copious narcotic resin. "Under the pressures of selection for these characters," Schultes wrote, "cannabis began to reveal characters and combinations of characters not found in wild or presumed wild populations, a phenomenon that has occurred in every plant domesticated by man."[15]

CANNABINOIDS: THE CANNABIS PLANT'S LITTLE MIRACLES

Perhaps the cannabis plant's most distinguishing feature, and a major source of its magic, is the presence of cannabinoids, active chemical components in the resin glands that plug into special receptors in the human brain and body to down regulate the nervous and immune systems, influencing appetite, pain sensation, inflammation, temperature regulation, muscle control, metabolism, stress response, mood, and memory. Robert C. Clarke and Mark D. Merlin suggest that cannabinoids—so rare that they can't be found even in cannabis's closest cousin, hops—exist solely to attract humans and other animals as an adaptive survival measure.[16] Researchers have isolated more than ninety cannabinoids since 1964, when Israeli scientist Dr. Raphael Mechoulam discovered the most famous cannabinoid, delta-9-tetrahydrocannabinol, or THC—the one that gets people high.

THC triggers CB1 receptors that determine how people see, smell, listen, and feel hunger, pleasure, and pain, as well as CB2 receptors in the liver, heart, kidneys, blood vessels, endocrine glands, and lymph cells, which modulate inflammation and pain. It induces mild reverie and euphoria; heightens sensory awareness, creativity, and empathy; impairs short-term memory; alters sense of time and space; enhances appetite and sexual desire; occasionally causes drowsiness; and has a tendency to enhance introspection.[17]

Cannabis is best known—both feared and loved—for the psychoactive properties of THC, but the plant contains plenty of other cannabinoids—cannabidiol (CBD), cannabinolic acid (CBN), cannabigerolic acid (CBG), cannabichromenic acid (CBCA), and cannabinodiolic acid (CBNDA) are a few—that scientists are just beginning to study. CBD has received the most scrutiny, and attention, because it presents a large array of pharmacological properties and is able to mitigate some of THC's negative side effects.

In 1992, Mechoulam made another big breakthrough in understanding the cannabis plant when he found naturally occurring cannabis-like molecules in the human body that maintain bodily homeostasis, or biological harmony in response to environmental changes, by modulating the flow of neurotransmitters to provide balance to all other systems. Mechoulam and his team realized the phytocannabinoids in cannabis (*phyto* means "of the plant") mimicked endocannabinoids (*endo* means "within"), which were one of the body's most widespread and versatile signaling molecules, affecting pain, memory, mood, appetite, stress, sleep, metabolism, and immune and reproductive functions. Phytocannabinoids stimulate and block CB receptors just like endocannabinoids do.

The two most common and well-understood endocannabinoids are anandamide (named after the Sanskrit word for "bliss"), which is similar in structure and function to THC, and 2-arachidonoylglycerol (2-AG), which acts much like CBD. THC attaches to what is known as an orthosteric binding site on the CB1 receptor in the same way that anandamide does, and CBD hooks up to an allosteric binding site on the same receptor, which reduces THC's psychoactive and other negative side effects such as tachycardia, anxiety, dysphoria, and depersonalization. CBD slows anandamide breakdown while increasing 2-AG production, which enhances the endocannabinoids' effects and creates what is known in the medical community as "endocannabinoid tone."

In 2004, Ethan B. Russo published a paper exploring the idea that clinical endocannabinoid deficiency (CECD) could be an underlying factor in migraines, fibromyalgia, irritable bowel syndrome, and other functional conditions that are alleviated by cannabis use, and clinical experience has since proven his theory. CECD, which can be a congenital condition or the result of stress or injury, impairs and can even shut down the body's metabolic and regulatory processes. Russo and others have found that migraine, fibromyalgia, irritable bowel syndrome, and related conditions display common clinical, biochemical, and pathophysiological patterns that suggest a clinical endocannabinoid deficiency is the underlying cause, and that deficiency could be treated with phytocannabinoids from cannabis.[18]

If medical researchers can figure out how to modulate the endocannabinoid system, it would open up a whole new world of therapeutic potential affecting almost every disease known to disrupt human health, including obesity; diabetes; neurodegenerative, inflammatory,

Major Cannabinoids in Cannabis

Tetrahydrocannabinol (THC): Reduces nausea and vomiting; relieves pain; stimulates appetite; suppresses muscle spasms
Cannabidiol (CBD): Antibacterial, neuroprotective, immunosuppressant, anti-inflammatory; inhibits cancer cell growth; promotes bone growth; reduces seizures and convulsions; relieves vomiting and nausea, pain and anxiety
Cannabichromene (CBC): Anti-inflammatory; inhibits cancer cell growth; promotes bone growth; relieves pain
Cannabigerol (CBG): Aids sleep; inhibits cancer cell growth; promotes bone growth; slows bacterial growth

Source: CertifiedMarijuanaDoctors.com

cardiovascular, liver, gastrointestinal, and skin diseases; pain; psychiatric disorders; cachexia; cancer; and chemotherapy-induced nausea.[19] "The endocannabinoid system is very important. Almost all illnesses we have are linked to it in some way or another," Mechoulam told *Vice* in 2016. "And that is very strange. We don't have many systems which get involved with every illness."[20]

TERPENES: "THE WORLD'S MOST SPOKEN LANGUAGE"

Cannabis gets its strong aroma and flavor from terpenes, highly volatile isoprene units that send out signals to attract pollinators, shoo away predators, and act as key agents in metabolic processes. Terpenes diffuse easily into the air and act as pheromones, communicating signals to other plants and insects to either retreat or come play. Netherlands Institute of Ecology researchers found that terpenes are "the most popular chemical medium on our planet to communicate through," leading them to give terpenes the poetic title, "the world's most spoken language."[21]

Terpenes can be found in all aromatic plants—bunya pines, for example, exude the terpene limonene in their latex to sound an alarm that keeps termites away, and ponderosa pines put out sap containing the terpene myrcene, which is toxic for invasive bark beetles—but with as many as 260 different terpenes (and still counting), cannabis has the richest and most robust patois of all plants.

For centuries, terpenes have been the treasured secret ingredient in the volatile oils used to make medicine, perfume, and cosmetics. In Aristotle's time, terpenes were so highly regarded that they were considered the quintessential fifth element or life force. Not only were they pleasing to the nose, but the aromatic oils were also found to bring about different moods and therapeutic effects when humans inhaled and consumed them.

In a groundbreaking 1993 paper, Dr. Ethan B. Russo stated that terpenes' interactions with the cannabinoids in cannabis "could produce synergy with respect to treatment of pain, inflammation, depression, anxiety, addiction, epilepsy, cancer, fungal and bacterial infections" while acting as "putative antidotes" to the intoxicating effects of THC.[22] Russo called this

Cannabis Terpenes

Beta-Caryophyllene
- **Aroma:** Pepper, cloves
- **Effects:** Calming, relaxing
- **High in Caryophyllene:** Super Silver Haze, Trainwreck

Borneol
- **Aroma:** Earthy, camphor
- **Effects:** Pain relief, sedative
- **High in Borneol:** Haze strains

Eucalyptol
- **Aroma:** Spicy, mint
- **Effects:** Calming, balancing
- **High in Eucalyptol:** Super Silver Haze

Limonene
- **Aroma:** Citrus
- **Effects:** Uplifting, euphoric
- **High in Limonene:** OG Kush, Super Lemon Haze

Linalool
- **Aroma:** Floral, sweet
- **Effects:** Sedative, relieves anxiety
- **High in Linalool:** Amnesia Haze

Myrcene
- **Aroma:** Musky, earthy
- **Effects:** Sedating, relaxing
- **High in Myrcene:** White Widow

Pinene
- **Aroma:** Pine
- **Effects:** Clarity, counteracts some THC effects
- **High in Pinene:** Super Silver Haze, Jack Herer, Trainwreck

Terpineol
- **Aroma:** Sweet, floral
- **Effects:** Relaxing, sedative
- **High in Terpineol:** Jack Herer

the "entourage effect," and his theory that cannabis offers superior benefits when all of its more than 480 natural components are left intact—that the plant's whole is superior to the sum of its parts—is now widely accepted in the cannabis and scientific communities.

Earlier humans may not have known to call them terpenes or understood the science behind them, but people have understood that these chemicals could moderate THC's psychoactive effects since at least the first century. Writing about cannabis in *Natural History, Book XXIV*, Pliny the Elder described a method for counteracting the effects of ingesting too much psychoactive THC with peppercorns—a trick that survived well into the twenty-first century. "The gelotophyllis ['leaves of laughter' = cannabis] grows in Bactria and along the Borysthenes," Pliny wrote. "If this be taken in myrrh and wine all kinds of phantoms beset the mind, causing laughter which persists until the kernels of pine nuts are taken with pepper and honey in palm wine."[23] (Twenty centuries later, rock star Neil Young would share that trick on air with radio shock jock Howard Stern.)

Russo deconstructed Pliny's overconsumption antidote in an article about the entourage effect, explaining that black pepper was effective because it offered mental clarity from the terpene pinene, sedation via myrcene, and helpful contributions from B-caryophyllene—a terpene so powerful that many believe it should be classified as a cannabinoid. "The historical suggestions for cannabis antidotes are thus supported by modern scientific rationale for the claims," Russo wrote, "and if proven experimentally would provide additional evidence of synergy."[24]

HEMP: THE VEGETABLE KINGDOM'S MOST MISUNDERSTOOD PLANT

The nutritious seeds of the hemp plant have been an important food source since the dawn of humans. Traditionally eaten as a staple food by people in the lower classes, the seeds carried multitudes of Chinese peasants through times of famine. Ancient Europeans spent long, arduous hours making a gritty peanut butter–type preparation by crushing the hulled seeds with their hands.

Thanks to modern seed dehulling technology invented in the twentieth century, the hemp seed available to consumers today is far superior to anything Chinese or European peasants could have prepared. Unfortunately, in most of the world hemp was prohibited alongside THC-rich marijuana in the 1930s. "Surely no member of the vegetable kingdom has ever been more misunderstood than hemp," David P. West wrote in a special report for the North American Industrial Hemp Council in 1998. "And nowhere have emotions run hotter than the debate over the distinction between industrial hemp and marijuana."[25]

Though they serve vastly different functions, do not look alike, and are often referred to as "cousins," industrial hemp and psychoactive "marijuana" are actually the same plant, *Cannabis sativa*, bred and cultivated in very different ways. For centuries, cannabis farmers have understood that when cannabis plants grow very close together, they get less sunlight and produce longer fiber-producing stems and no psychoactive resin. To produce plants full of sticky flowers, farmers sow seeds farther apart to give each plant more sunlight; the plants secrete more resin to protect themselves from drying out.[26]

In determining the difference between the two, which became increasingly important as stricter drug laws were enacted worldwide in the late 1960s and early 1970s, Canadian researcher Ernest Small somewhat randomly stated that plants could be called hemp if they had less than 0.3 percent THC. This definition would become the internationally accepted standard and was written into most of the legislation outlawing marijuana in the 1970s.

Hemp cultivation was made illegal in North America because of "concern that the hemp crop was a drug menace," Small wrote in a 2002 paper. The United States, the European Community, and Canada used Small's 0.3 percent THC content as a dividing line between "cultivars that can be legally cultivated under license and forms that are considered to have too high a drug potential."

Small's paper explained that there was a general inverse relationship in cannabis resin between the amount of THC present and the amount of the other principal cannabinoid, CBD. Whereas most strains used as drugs contained primarily THC and little or no CBD, the cultivars bred for fiber and oilseed primarily contained CBD and very little THC[27]—they could not get anyone high, no matter how much they imbibed. This distinction would continue to be very important when CBD emerged as a medical and therapeutic agent and functional food in the 2000s, and many states and countries approved its use well before they made cannabis containing THC legal.

In 1999, the United States began allowing the import of hemp products with less than 0.3 percent THC, and in the 2010s it began allowing limited domestic cultivation of industrial hemp, which was being used to make everything from food and body care products to insulation. As more consumers embraced hemp foods and demand for CBD surged, more states established hemp programs and production soared in the United States.

Between 2016 and 2017, the number of hemp producers doubled, and the number of acres licensed for hemp cultivation in the top ten hemp-growing states grew by 140 percent.[28] In 2018, Republican Senate Majority Leader Mitch McConnell submitted a bill to unshackle hemp from its illicit "cousin" by removing it from the federal government's list of controlled substances. "First and foremost," he said, "this bill will finally legalize hemp as an agricultural commodity."[29]

CANNABIS: A NUTRITIONAL POWERHOUSE

Primitive humans followed good instincts when they began cultivating cannabis as a food source.

The soft, white kernels inside cannabis seeds' hard shell produce high-protein oil high in essential fatty acids (EFAs), phosphorous, potassium, magnesium, sulfur, calcium, iron, zinc, carotene (a precursor to vitamin A), tocopherols (major antioxidants that include the vitamin E group),[30] thiamin (vitamin B1), riboflavin (vitamin B2), vitamin B6, chlorophyll, sulfur, phosphorus, phosphosolipids, and phytosterols. Cannabis is the only current natural food source of gamma-linolenic acid (GLA), which affects vital metabolic roles ranging from control of inflammation and vascular tone to hormone balancing.

Cannabis seeds have extremely low THC content and taste creamy and nutty, without the bitterness of the plant material. They can be shelled and eaten like sunflower seeds or ground into a powder for snacking and cooking. They're high in roughage and easily digestible edestin protein, which is likely why they became a staple for healing digestive issues in Traditional Chinese Medicine and other healing modalities. The seeds' ideal 1:3 ratio of omega-3 and omega-6 EFAs provides more of these compounds—which are called "essential" because they must come from a source outside the body—than fish. They're high in linoleic acid and alpha-linolenic acid, which are difficult to come by in Western diets and act as raw materials for cell structure and as biosynthesis precursors for many of the body's regulatory biochemicals.

The raw cannabis plant does not contain actual cannabinoids, but it does contain cannabinoid acids that must be activated, usually through heat, to unleash their therapeutic properties. Heating cannabis to about 200 degrees Fahrenheit breaks off THC-A's and CBD-A's carboxyl radicals and converts them to THC and CBD through a process called decarboxylation. This is why people smoke or vaporize cannabis and why chefs often toast it in the oven before cooking with it.

Because THC, CBD, and other cannabinoids, as well as terpenes, are fat soluble, they bind with fats such as oil, butter, or milk when heated. Alcohol also works to extract cannabinoids and terpenes. When cooking with cannabis, chefs throughout the ages have made extractions, pulling cannabinoids from the leaves and flowers by heating them gently in a fat, then straining out the plant matter. Simmering the cannabis and oil or butter over low heat for anywhere from thirty minutes to several days allows the cannabinoids and terpenes time to infuse into the medium, but the temperature must never get high enough to evaporate them.

Tinctures made with alcohol have also been a time-tested method of extracting and preserving cannabinoids and terpenes, and most Americans consumed cannabis in over-the-counter tinctures until Prohibition began in 1937. Alcohol softens and separates the cannabis in a process called maceration, which can take from six hours to ten days. Heating the infusion hastens the extraction.

Eating cannabis is an entirely different process of delivering cannabinoids to the bloodstream than smoking it and produces very divergent effects. When cannabis is smoked or vaped, delta-9 THC enters the bloodstream through the lungs within fifteen minutes. When it's eaten, it is broken down with acid and enzymes in the stomach before being sent through the liver, where another step is added before cannabinoids enter the bloodstream. The liver converts delta-9 THC into 11-hydroxy-THC, which crosses the blood-brain barrier more rapidly and, for most people, delivers a much more potent and longer-lasting high.

Fatty, protein-rich foods intensify THC's effects, sugar creates a faster high that dissipates more quickly, and alcohol can compound the effects and induce anxiety or paranoia. A complicated set of variables also factor into how long it takes for cannabis to hit a person's system and how strongly it affects them, including the individual's age, metabolism, body size and mass, personal biochemistry, age, and tolerance, as well as how the food and infusion were prepared and the food it's combined with.

RAW CANNABIS: "A UNIQUE FUNCTIONAL FOOD"

When cannabis is eaten raw, as the cavepeople did, it is a digestible complete protein that provides essential amino acids and omega fatty acids, as well as the plant kingdom's largest source of cannabinoids. Technically a fruit because of its seed-bearing flowers, raw cannabis is a nutritional powerhouse that has been largely ignored since humans discovered that heating the flowers or finding another way of extracting the plant's resin heightens its psychoactive and therapeutic effects.

When cannabis is heated to convert its carboxylic acids into cannabinoids (decarboxylation), the plant's chemical composition is altered as well. The process actually strips out some cannabinoids and terpenes, with all their beneficial antioxidant and anti-inflammatory properties, too. Dr. William Courtney, a Mendocino County physician who recommends that his patients eat raw cannabis flowers or juice raw cannabis every day to maximize the plant's health benefits, states that heating THC reduces the total antioxidant dose it delivers to one-fiftieth of what it was when the plant was raw. "The biggest drawback to steeping, sautéing, baking, smoking, or vaporizing cannabis is that the THC generated creates a marked reduction in the THC-A/CBD-A dosage," Courtney wrote in a journal article, "Cannabis as a Unique Functional Food."[31]

Courtney's domestic partner, Kristen Peskuski, successfully treated lupus, interstitial cystitis, and rheumatoid arthritis using a regimen of eating fifteen cannabis leaves and two large flowers every day. Courtney said the extensive number of patents that have been granted for cannabinoids and a growing body of scientific evidence convinced him that cannabis could have a remediating effect on diabetes, cancer, autoimmune disorders, and ischemic conditions and qualify for recognition as Essential Cannabinoid Acids across the entire lifespan—but only if eaten raw. "Cannabis, a unique functional food if used in its natural state, daily, provides benefits in excess of nutrition," Courtney stated.[32]

Eating raw cannabis will not get most people stoned because the THC-A has not been converted to psychoactive THC. Ethnobotanist and Medicine Hunter Chris Kilham said he has gotten plenty high while eating raw cannabis with indigenous people around the world, however, and he dared anyone to disagree.

"If you eat cannabinoids, you get an effect," Kilham said. "Eating raw cannabis is an old, common method. Eat cannabis, get high."

FAN LEAVES: SYMBOLS OF THE TIMES

The pointy fan leaf has been a symbol for cannabis culture and an enduring icon since the earliest humans began enjoying cannabis. The oldest depiction found so far dates to the Neolithic era and was painted on a cave wall on the coast of Kyushu, Japan. In ancient Egypt, many historians believe, people painted a plant with pointy leaves above the head of Seshat, goddess of architecture, astronomy, astrology, and mathematics, to communicate cannabis's revelatory aspects.

In the nineteenth and early twentieth centuries, when cannabis was a common ingredient in over-the-counter elixirs in the United States, the fan leaf was often represented on medicine bottle labels. It went underground with the advent of Prohibition in 1937, largely forgotten until it reemerged, along with tie dye and peace signs, in the antiauthority 1960s. At the height of its newfound popularity, Gram Parsons had suits with cannabis leaves embroidered on them made for him and his Flying Burrito Brothers bandmates to wear on the cover of their first album in 1969.

In the 1980s, as hippies became yuppies, the leaf went back underground, and then it went corporate. Adidas drew the wrath of the US drug czar in 1998 when it replaced its logo with a cannabis leaf to market sports shoes made from hemp. As prohibition laws were relaxed and public opinion grew more favorable to cannabis in the 2010s, the leaf became a no-longer-avant-garde icon that could be spotted everywhere from fashion runways to Jacquie Aiche Sweet Leaf jewelry (a favorite of A-listers) to the logos of countless companies jumping into the newly legal cannabis industry.

Cannabis sativa, in Slang

There have been at least 1,200 slang terms for cannabis and hundreds more to describe the intoxicated state it induces throughout history, according to *Time* magazine. Slang scholar Jonathon Green, who kept a database of worldwide argots and their origins, explained that people develop code words as a means of protection when they're doing something criminal but also because it's "seen as fighting the man" and it's "simply fun."[1] Green said the word *pot*, which was synonymous with cannabis in the late twentieth and early twenty-first centuries, came from *potiguaya*, which is Mexican Spanish for cannabis leaves. He first came across the use of the commonly used word *weed* in reference to cannabis in a 1904 *Indianapolis News* clipping.[2]

The following are slang terms that have been used for cannabis, from various times and places.

420
alfalfa
Amsterdam's Finest
asparagus
Aunt Mary
bammy
BC
bhang
blunt
bone
bongo
boo
bud
Buddha
cabbage
Caracas
catnip
charas
cheeba
Cheech and Chong
choke
Christmas tree
chronic
grass

Colorado Cocktail
crop
dagga
dank
delta-9
Detroit
devil's lettuce
diesel
Dona Juanita
doobage
dope
dro
dutchie
endo
fatty
flower
frodis
funk
gage
ganja
giggle stick
goddess
grade
nugs

green
Green Goddess
gwaai
hash
hay
headies
hemp
herb
hierba
hippie lettuce
Houdini
hydro
Indian hay
Indo
Jane
jazz cabbage
Jimmy
keef
kibbies
kif
kind bud
Kush
laughing grass
loco weed
love weed
marijuana
Mary
Mary Jane
mezz
mids
morning meds
moss
mota
muggles
outdo
pakololo
pocket rocket
pot
purp
rainy day woman
reefer
reggs
rope
schwag
Scooby Doo
sinse
Sister Mary
skunk
smoke
spliff
stank
stash
sticky icky
sweet leaf
Sweet Lucy
tacos
taima
tea
trees
tweed
viper
wacky tobaccy
weed
wheat
Yellow Submarine
yerba
yuyo
zacate

NOTES

1. Katy Steinmetz, "420 Day: Why There Are So Many Different Names for Weed," Time.com, April 20, 2017, http://time.com/4747501/420-day-weed-marijuana-pot-slang/.

2. Jak Hutchcraft, "The Roots of Cannabis Slang," Prohbtd.com, October 22, 2017, https://prohbtd.com/the-roots-of-cannabis-slang.

Cannabis: A Brief History

600 BC: The Scythians use cannabis in vapor baths. Greek historian Herodotus later writes that they "enjoy it so much they howl with pleasure."

AD 70: Greek physician and Roman army doctor Pedanius Dioscorides includes cannabis as a cure for earaches and overripe libido in *De Materia Medica.*

79: Pliny the Elder writes in *Naturalis Historia* that cannabis roots boiled in water "ease cramped joints, gout too and similar violent pain."

168: People in China's Hunan province use cannabis for religious, medicinal, and divination purposes.

1100s: Hassan-ibn-Sabbah, the Old Man of the Mountain, rules the *Hashshashin* (Assassins) in northern Persia by feeding them a hashish-based confection known as *majoun* (sometimes *majoon*). Majoun is popular in India, along with a drink made from cannabis called *bhang* and hashish known as *charas*.

1155: Sufi master Sheik Haydar writes that he has invented hashish.

1273: Marco Polo writes about the Old Man of the Mountain in accounts of his journeys through Persia.

1378: Ottoman Sultan Nigm al din Ayoub issues an edict that anyone caught growing cannabis or eating hashish will have their teeth pulled.

1475: The world's first printed cookbook, *On Honourable Pleasure and Health* by Bartolomeo Platina, includes a recipe for "a health drink of cannabis nectar."

1484: Pope Innocent VIII declares cannabis use cause for excommunication.

1600s: Hashish is a major trade item between Central Asia and South Asia.

1619: Virginia Assembly requires every farmer to grow hemp. Hemp is exchanged as legal tender in Pennsylvania, Virginia, and Maryland.

1753: Swedish botanist Carl Linnaeus introduces *Cannabis sativa* in his *Species Plantarum.*

1798: Napoleon's occupation of Egypt brings hashish to Paris. Napoleon prohibits hashish use.

1830s: Irish physician William Brooke O'Shaughnessy discovers cannabis during a trip to India and introduces it to colleagues as a means to treat muscle spasms, rheumatism, epilepsy, and pain.

1840s: Queen Victoria's personal physician, Sir Robert Russell, recommends cannabis tinctures for menstrual cramps.

1844–1849: Writers, artists, and musicians in Paris form the *Club des Hashischins* (Club of the Hashish-Eaters).

1850: Cannabis is added to the US Pharmacopeia for ailments including neuralgia, tetanus, typhus, cholera, rabies, dysentery, alcoholism, opiate addiction, anthrax, leprosy, incontinence, gout, convulsive disorders, tonsillitis, insanity, excessive menstrual bleeding, and uterine bleeding.

1857: *The Hasheesh Eater: Being Passages from the Life of Pythagorean*, by Fitz Hugh Ludlow, is published.

1860s–1900s: Gunjah Wallah hashish–based maple candies are popular in the United States.

1900: The Indian *Materia Medica* lists cannabis as an important drug, used for asthma, bronchitis, and loss of appetite.

1910: Mexican immigrants fleeing the Mexican Revolution bring recreational cannabis use to the United States.

1911: Massachusetts is the first state to outlaw cannabis.

1913: California and Jamaica outlaw cannabis.

1917: George Schlichten invents the decorticator, dramatically reducing the labor required to separate hemp fibers from stalks.

1920s: Marijuana clubs, known as "tea pads," operate in every major US city.

1925: The League of Nations restricts cannabis use to scientific and medical purposes and places restrictions on importing and exporting.

1937: Propaganda film *Reefer Madness* is released. The Marihuana Tax Act makes recreational use of marijuana illegal but allows physicians and pharmacists who pay an annual tax or license fee to prescribe and dispense it.

1938: Canada bans cannabis cultivation.

1942: Cannabis is removed from the US Pharmacopeia.

1954: *The Alice B. Toklas Cook Book*, containing a recipe for Hashish Fudge, is published.

1961: International treaty the Single Convention on Narcotic Drugs prohibits production and supply of drugs, including cannabis.

1964: Israeli chemist Dr. Raphael Mechoulam identifies THC as cannabis's main psychoactive component and is the first to synthesize THC.

1966: *The Hashish Cookbook*, by Panama Rose, is published.

1968: *I Love You, Alice B. Toklas!*, the first major motion picture to use cannabis as an important part of the plot, is released.

1970: The Controlled Substances Act makes marijuana a Schedule 1 drug, equivalent to heroin, with no medical uses. National Organization for the Reform of Marijuana Laws is founded.

1972: Mellow Yellow, the first coffee shop in Amsterdam, opens.
1976: The Netherlands decriminalizes cannabis.
1988: San Francisco voters overwhelmingly pass Proposition P, restoring hemp medical preparations to the list of available medicines in California. *High Times* hires Chef Ra to write a monthly cannabis food column.
1992: The country's first public medical cannabis dispensary, the Cannabis Buyers' Club, opens in San Francisco.
1996: California voters pass Proposition 215, permitting the sale and use of medical marijuana.
2001: Spain's first cannabis social club, *Club de Catadores*, opens in Barcelona.
2009: US Deputy Attorney General David W. Ogden releases memo declaring the federal government will not go after patients who use cannabis for cancer or other serious illnesses.
2012: Voters in Colorado and Washington approve measures legalizing adult use of cannabis.
2013: Uruguay is the first country to legalize and regulate adult use of cannabis.
2014: Colorado and Washington create the world's first legal cannabis markets.
2015: Jamaica decriminalizes cannabis, legalizes medical marijuana, and makes it legal for Jamaicans to grow five plants per household.
2016: Voters in California, the world's fifth-largest economy, legalize adult use of cannabis.
2018: Canada legalizes adult use of cannabis.

• 2 •

Food of the Ancients

The Chinese were the first people to domesticate cannabis, most historians believe, initially as food and then as a fiber source. During the Neolithic period in China, as the Yangshao culture transitioned from hunting and gathering to nomadic agriculture, picking up and moving on once they had depleted the soil, communities flourished along the loess plains of the Huang He (Yellow River) by cultivating millet and some wheat and rice as subsistence crops alongside hemp, which they used to make rope, clothing, sails, and bowstrings (see photo on next page). The Yangshao people were so enamored with cannabis that they decorated their famous red-painted pottery with pictures of it.

In the Chinese written language, cannabis's character, *ma*, depicts hemp stalks hanging to dry, and it has two meanings—"numerous or chaotic," which is derived from the way hemp fibers are tangled together, and "numbness or senselessness," referring to the effects of using the flowers in medical preparations[1]—indicating that both industrial hemp and narcotic strains of the *Cannabis sativa* plant have been used since writing began. The Chinese were no strangers to the mind-altering effects of the cannabis plant's resinous leaves and flowers, but most people in China were never too sure about whether that should be considered a benefit or a hazard. They called cannabis both "the liberator of sin" and "the delight giver."[2]

In the folklore about cannabis that's been handed down through the ages, proof of its use and popularity as medicine is often attributed to two mythical deities. A pharmacist named Shen Nung was said to write about the plant in his pharmacopeia (long before paper

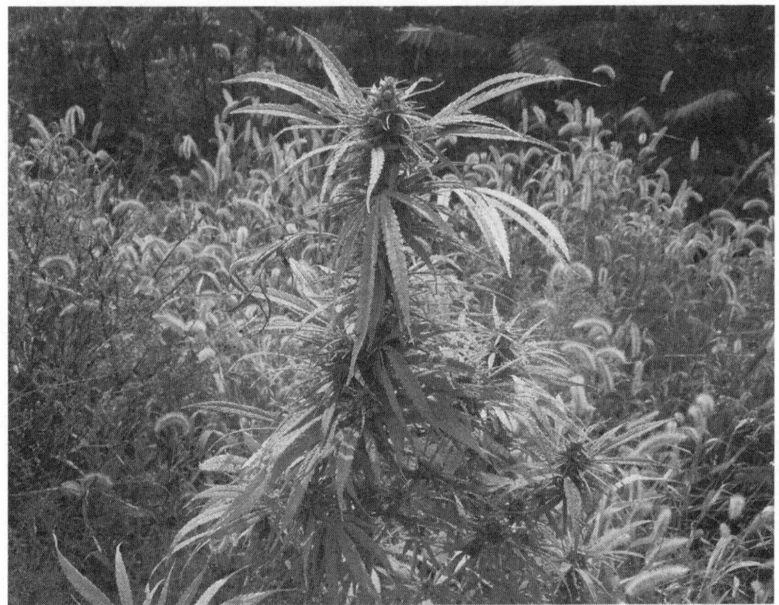

Cannabis growing in China's Xinjian region along the ancient Silk Road trade route. Photo by Chris Kilham.

was invented) in 2737 BCE. Another tall tale attributes Emperor Fu, the telepathic, wild-animal-taming fictional first emperor of China, with saying that *ma* was a popular medicine in China because it possessed both yin and yang, giving it the ability to both relax and enliven people. These urban legends became so widely accepted as fact that they were written into many history books and cited by reputable sources.

What we do know for fact is that throughout ancient history, and once paper was invented, Chinese texts recommended ingesting hemp seed for urinary and blood flow problems, palsy, breast milk production, muscle fiber growth, dysentery, and constipation.[3] In a rare reference to the plant's psychoactive and hallucinogenic effects in the fifth century CE, a Taoist priest wrote in the *Ming-I Pieh Lu* that necromancers used cannabis in combination with ginseng "to set forward time in order to reveal future events." For the most part, however, cannabis's mind-altering properties were not documented and remained a shadowy, closely held secret among the indigenous shamans of central Asia.[4]

The transition from hunter-gatherer to farming culture was a good one for the Chinese people. By the time of the Western Zhou dynasty (1021 to 771 BCE), the masses had grown affluent and could feed themselves well. Cannabis seeds were one of their most important "cereals" along with millet and buckwheat.[5] For centuries, until it was superseded by other grains such as soybeans and rice, cannabis was an indispensable component in Chinese peasants' diets. Many poor people subsisted on a porridge made from ground cannabis seeds, but they were hardly the only ones to appreciate cannabis's benefits as a high-protein, well-balanced food.

In the twenty-first century, archaeologists found containers of hemp seeds among the agricultural products in the tomb of an elite woman who died a few years after 168 CE at Ma-wang-tui on the eastern outskirts of Changsha in Hunan province. Archaeologists have unearthed evidence of cannabis use from sites throughout the country. Cannabis fruits, leaves, and shoots were found along with caper seeds in a pottery jar, which was likely used for religious or medicinal purposes, dating to 2700 BP in the Yanghai Tombs near Turpan, Xinjiang-Uyghur Autonomous Region. The grave of a Caucasoid shaman found in the same tombs included a large cache of THC-containing cannabis that most likely was used as a psychoactive agent or a tool to aid in divination.[6]

Some historians believe early Taoists in China combined cannabis with other ingredients to make elixirs that they consumed during fervent religious ceremonies that were often associated with the Hemp Maid, or *Ma Gu*,[7] but "the Chinese experiment with marihuana as a psychoactive agent was really more of a flirtation than an orgy," E. L. Abel wrote in *Marihuana: The First Twelve Thousand Years*. "Those among the Chinese who hailed it as the 'giver of delight' never amounted to more than a small segment of the population."

Taoists eventually came to disdain cannabis because they believed it induced yin energy (negative, dark, and feminine), and they favored only substances that filled them with yang (positive, bright, and masculine). Cannabis would continue to be used as food and medicine, but its mind-altering properties were, for the most part, considered a side effect rather than a benefit.

INDIA: "LENGTHENER OF LIFE, FREER FROM THE BONDS OF SELF"

Perhaps more than anywhere else in the world, cannabis has been an integral part of health, recreation, and spiritual life as well as a key component to many archetypal origin stories in India.

It all begins with an ancient Indian folk legend from the highlands in which an angry servant invites tigers and bears as well as snakes and scorpions—who, back in those days, stood upright and looked humans in the eye—to attend a wedding being sponsored by a sorcerer who had mistreated her when she worked for him. The tigers and bears were more than happy to drink pot after pot of the sorcerer's fine liquor, but the snakes and scorpions demanded *ganja*, which was the name for cannabis flowers from the Ganges Mountains.

The sorcerer was a drinker, not a smoker, and he had no ganja. Growing concerned as his venomous guests grew restless, the sorcerer pulled two leaves from the hallucinogenic datura plant and rubbed them

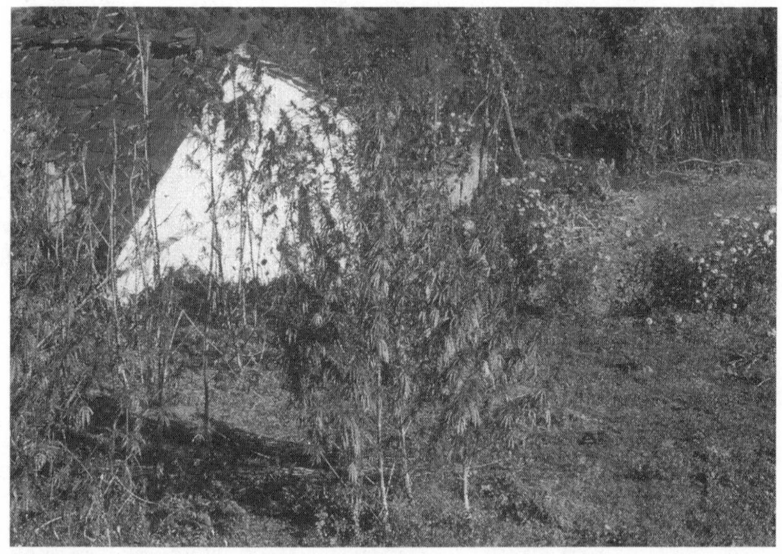

Cannabis growing in India's Ranikhet region in the Himalayas. Photo by Chris Kilham.

together until a drop of juice fell to the ground. In that moment, the first cannabis plant was born. The sorcerer mixed juice from that plant with water, filled a pipe, and gave it to the snakes and scorpions, who laughed and danced with such intoxicated abandon that they broke their backs and fell to the ground, where they were doomed to slither on the ground forevermore.

Archeologists believe a group of Aryan warrior-nomads brought cannabis to South Asia during a series of invasions between 2000 and 1000 BCE, and it became a critical part of the culture, used in religious rituals and festivals, ingested as medicine, and enjoyed recreationally—though in very different forms—by people from all castes. Ancient Sanskrit poems celebrate cannabis as one of five kingdoms of herbs that release people from anxiety, and the Hindu scripture *Bhagavad Gita* sings its praises, saying cannabis can sharpen memory and alleviate fatigue.

Siddhartha, the wealthy, young prince who sat under a Bodhi tree for six years preparing for spiritual enlightenment, was said to eat nothing but a single cannabis seed per day during his incubation to become the Buddha. The *Atharva Veda*, a Hindu scripture written between 2000 and 1400 BCE, referred to cannabis as an ingredient in an intoxicating drink called *soma*, and ancient Hindu poetry is filled with references to how Lord Shiva, one of three gods responsible for creating, maintaining, and destroying the world, loved cannabis so much that he brought the plant from the Himalayas as his gift to humankind.

The earliest practitioners of Ayurvedic medicine were convinced that cannabis could soothe the fevers that plagued humankind, which Lord Shiva was said to have blown from his nostrils during a fit of anger at his father-in-law, Prajapati, the king of all men. (Later on in the mythical tales, Lord Shiva killed Daksha.) Ancient Indians called cannabis *vijaya*, which in the Sanskrit language meant "victorious," and it was widely believed that Lord Shiva gave it to humans as a gift because he was concerned about the welfare of all people.

Though cannabis use was widespread throughout India, methods of consuming it were very different and determined, as was most everything in the culture, by the caste system that divides Hindu society into hereditary classes. The higher castes made the leaves and flowers into a paste known as *bhang*, which was usually combined with spices, seeds, nuts, and milk to make a creamy drink called *Bhang ki Thandai* (a name generally shortened to bhang) and was consumed during religious rites and celebrations. Throughout the centuries, Indian writers have waxed poetic about the many benefits of bhang, which they have described as an exhilarating substance that stimulated conversation, eager thought, and poetic imagination; induced sleep and sexual desire; increased fertility; and cured diseases.

The celebratory beverage was traditionally prepared by pounding and mixing the leaves with water to form a thick paste, which was then rolled into a ball and allowed to dry. The dried paste was then mixed with milk to solubilize the fat-soluble THC, strained through a cloth, mixed with more milk or water, and flavored with sugar, spices such as cardamom and ginger, and sometimes melon seeds.

By the twelfth century CE, bhang had become a mandatory gesture of hospitality for many Indians as well as the drink of warriors, who often took a swig to build courage and calm their nerves before they marched into battle. In a famous legend, Guru Gobind Singh, who founded the Sikh religion, is said to have given panicked soldiers bhang and opium when he saw them wavering during a critical battle. Once the drugs kicked in, Singh watched, mesmerized, as one intrepid soldier stabbed an elephant in the belly to kill it. Singh's men won the battle, and they celebrated by drinking, of course, bhang.[8]

Throughout India, use of cannabis and public approval or disapproval of its consumption varied, nearly always based on caste position. The elite castes in Madras consumed a lot of bhang, while the laboring poor in Hyderabad and *fakirs* (religious ascetics) in Delhi, who couldn't afford bhang, made do with ganja, which was prepared from the flowering tops of cultivated female cannabis plants. Harvard Medical School psychiatrist and cannabis researcher Lester Grinspoon likened the difference between ganja and bhang to the variation between beer, the drink of commoners, and fine single-malt scotch, a liquor for elites.

Sometimes lower-caste Hindus pressed sticky cannabis resin into balls or wafers known as *charas*, which was sold in measurements known as "fingers" and smoked in small pipes called *chillums*. Charas, because it was made from pure resin—which is where most of the THC is concentrated—was more psychoactively potent than bhang. It was also mixed with alcohol, perfumed syrups, and rose, jasmine, or orange water to make "exotic potions,"[9] and charas was a key ingredient in *majoun* (also spelled *majoon*), sweetmeats that were made from sesame seed oil, cocoa butter, spices, powdered chocolate, almonds, walnuts, pistachios, cinnamon, cloves, vanilla, musk, nutmeg, and belladonna berries[10]—confections that would become an enduring and important part of cannabis cultures around the world for centuries to come.

In India, majoun recipes varied from region to region and family to family, but nearly every family had one, and they were often closely guarded. Poppy seeds were often included, and sometimes so was datura, a leafy herb that causes uncomfortable and unpleasant effects including hallucinations, motor control loss, muscle spasms, and difficulty breathing. It was this powerful deliriant, not cannabis, that likely caused the extreme reactions to majoun that would tarnish the reputation of cannabis and hashish and be used as powerful propaganda against the plant for centuries.

In Ayurvedic medicine, one of the world's oldest medical systems, food was considered an integral component of optimal health. Ayurvedic physicians used cannabis as an important ingredient alongside other functional foods and spices in recipes designed to treat a variety of ailments and conditions. They believed that cannabis contained a warming energy or gastric fire called *pittala*, which they believed was one of three energies, or *doshas*, that circulated throughout the body and governed all physiological activity.

Cannabis was a trusted staple in most Ayurvedic doctors' arsenals, used to treat a wide range of health issues, most of them having to do with the nervous system and gastrointestinal tract, and relied upon as an aphrodisiac. *Jatiphaladi churna*, a remedy for diarrhea, indigestion, appetite loss, cough, and impotence, was made by mixing a mixture of nutmeg, cinnamon, ginger, cumin, cloves, cardamom, pepper, camphor, sandalwood, bamboo manna, sesame, *tejapatra* leaves, *Mesua ferrea* flowers, and all three myrobalans (*Terminalia chebula*, *T. bellerica*, and *Phyllanthus emblica* fruits) with bhang and sugar. Bhang, ghee (clarified butter), pepper, and poppy seeds were combined to treat diarrhea, and warm gingilie oil with bhang, onions, and turmeric was used as a salve for painful piles.[11]

When the British East India Company arrived to exploit Indian trade routes, labor, and resources in the mid-eighteenth century, most of the European merchants had never been exposed to cannabis. They couldn't help but notice how important bhang, ganja, and charas were to Indian people from all walks of life. Accordingly, they took control of the trade and taxed it heavily.

The new rulers created an agency that brought in considerable income from granting licenses to retailers and wholesalers who sold bhang, ganja, and charas, most of it made from cannabis produced in the fertile Ganges-Brahmaputra delta system in the Bengal region and shipped throughout India and into other parts of the empire. (When supplies ran low, more cannabis could always be brought from neighboring Turkestan, where it was also popular.) The British said the system of regulation was instituted "with a view to check immoderation consumption, and at the same time to augment the public revenue."[12] A government crackdown that imposed stringent restrictions on the sale and use of bhang and ganja made cannabis seem dangerous and gave it a criminal aura—and indeed, any cannabis cultivator who attempted to dodge the hefty British taxes and licensing fees was treated as an outlaw.

Though the colonialists tolerated cannabis use, they also condemned it and looked down upon Indians who used it. They based their opinions on plentiful British literature about the dangers associated with cannabis, much of it written by the day's most reputable sources, who repeated widespread rumors that lunatic asylums in India were overflowing with ganja smokers. A 1779 guide titled "Portable Instructions for Purchasing the Drugs and Spices of Asia and the East Indies" was a prime example of the type of propaganda that was distributed in India and throughout Europe. The pamphlet warned that bhang produced "a temporary madness, that in some, when designedly taken for that purpose, ends in running what they call a-muck, furiously killing every one they meet, without distinction, until themselves are knocked on the head, like mad dogs."[13] These reports would plant the seeds for a particularly effective form of propaganda claiming that cannabis was a menace to society, particularly threatening to youth, that propelled helpless users toward extreme violence and an unquenchable, uninhibited need to have sex—ideas that endured well into the twenty-first century.

In the 1830s, a well-respected Irish physician named William Brooke O'Shaughnessy traveled extensively throughout India and recorded his observations about health and medicine in the country, which was still considered exotic and even frightening to people back home. O'Shaughnessy observed that cannabis was widely used and, for the most part, he believed it was harmless. His writing about the plant's medical potential based on what he learned from Ayurvedic medical practitioners, particularly its anticonvulsive properties, stimulated renewed interest in the plant in Western medical circles. O'Shaughnessy fanned the flames of the already deeply rooted belief that cannabis users were potentially criminally insane, however, with descriptions of how cannabis could induce "a singular form of delirium."

Usually, O'Shaughnessy stated, cannabis induced cheerful inebriation and made users inclined to sing, dance, eat voraciously, and "seek aphrodisiac enjoyments." He also warned that it could put people into a unique and terrifying delirium, which could be "at once recognized by the strange balancing gait of the patient's; a constant rubbing of the hands; perpetual giggling; and a propensity to caress and chafe the feet of all bystanders of whatever rank. The eye wears an expression of cunning and merriment which can scarcely be mistaken. In a few cases, the patients are violent; in many highly aphrodisiac."[14] In the prudish Victorian era, that last suggestion was perhaps more appalling to O'Shaughnessy's readers than the threat of violence.

After the East India Company was dissolved and India formally came under direct British rule in 1858, the Indian people began to grow restless and resentful as the British Crown imposed iron-fisted rules of law and failed to respond adequately when the Bubonic plague swept the nation and killed millions. Though it would last for nearly another one hundred years, the India colony was already beginning to show signs of the tensions that would lead to its unraveling by the late nineteenth century. The colonialists, in need of a scapegoat as rumbles of disorder took root across the nation, blamed cannabis. As the propaganda campaign was amped up, fear and anticannabis sentiment ballooned, reaching all the way to the British House of Commons.

In 1893, the British Raj put together a special task force, the Indian Hemp Drug Commission, made up of four British and three Indian bureaucrats from a wide range of professions, to investigate cannabis use in India and recommend whether or not it should be prohibited. Between 1893 and 1894, the commissioners received evidence from 1,455 people across the country during field trips to thirty cities in eight provinces and Burma.[15] The commission's nine-volume report, looking at how cannabis use and culture affected and was affected by finance, trade, health, demography, crime, education, agriculture, history, and religion, was one of the most thoroughly investigated, comprehensive studies about cannabis that has ever been conducted. The report includes information about cultivation, preparation, trade and movement, consumption, social and religious customs, "moderation and excess," mental effects, and thorough examination of policies such as taxation, licensing, and prohibition.

The majority of the commission concluded that prohibiting ganja, charas, and bhang was "neither necessary nor expedient" because the hemp drugs were relatively harmless, consumption was limited, and they had social and religious significance. Not only was bhang essential to festivals such as Diwali, but it was an integral part of weddings and "merry family gatherings," the report stated.

Instead of prohibition, the commission recommended a policy of "control and restriction," which meant even more regulation and steeper taxes on cannabis, from cultivation licensing to retail taxes and restrictions on the amount people could possess—a policy that remained more or less intact well into the twentieth century. (Nearly a century later, in 1944, Asia expert Gertrude Emerson Sen wrote that she found hemp growing wild in every corner of the country during her travels in India but said she could not collect samples because the government restricted the right to collect and sell it.[16])

The seven members of the Hemp Drugs Commission were concerned that prohibition could drive consumers to take up more harmful drugs instead.

> By the help of bhang, ascetics pass days without food or drink. The supporting power of bhang has brought many a Hindu family safe through the miseries of famine. To forbid or even seriously to restrict the use of so holy and gracious a herb as the hemp would cause widespread suffering and annoyance and to large bands of worshipped ascetics, deep-seated anger, the report stated. It would rob the people of a solace in discomfort, of a cure in sickness, of a guardian whose gracious protection saves them from attacks of evil influences, and whose mighty power makes the devotee of the Victorious, overcoming the demons of hunger and thirst, of panic fear, of the glamour of Maya or matter, and of madness, able in rest to brood on the Eternal, til the Eternal, possessing him body and soul, frees him from the having of self and receives him into the ocean of Being. Those beliefs the Musalman devotee shares to the full. Like his Hindu brother the Musalman *fakir* reveres bhang as the lengthener of life, the freer from the bonds of self. Bhang brings union with the Divine Spirit. "We drank bhang and the mystery I am He grew plain." So grand a result, so tiny a sin![17]

Two of the three Indian members of the commission, who were from the "enlightened classes," wrote lengthy minority opinions that demonstrated the caste-based conflicts surrounding the different forms of cannabis use. The Indian commissioners called for absolute prohibition of ganja and charas—favorites of the lower castes—and absolute exemption of bhang—their own consumption method of choice—from control and restriction. "Intelligent and respectable Hindus" regarded ganja use as a vice, one dissenter wrote, adding that it was used chiefly by fakirs and the lower classes (artisans, cultivators, fishermen, *palki*-bearers, day laborers, and domestic servants).[18] The Indian commissioners also made no secret of their opinions that the British were motivated by the money they could make from taxing and licensing cannabis rather than acting for the good of the people in choosing to tax and control instead of instituting prohibition.

In an investigation that would reverberate well beyond the next century, the Indian Hemp Drugs Commission of 1893 spent considerable time and energy investigating the long-burning question, which had been debated in botanical circles since Lamarck's time, of whether "the narcotic-yielding plant is identical to the fibre-yielding plant."[19]

The commissioners surmised, quite presciently, that inquiring into the longstanding argument about whether *Cannabis indica* and *Cannabis sativa* were one species or two would be important in the future because of the possibility that "the restriction of the production of the narcotic by limiting the cultivation may affect a product and an industry which are above suspicion."

The commissioners based their conclusion on studies conducted by botanical researcher Dr. J. M. Watt, who wrote: "*Cannabis indica* has been reduced to *Cannabis sativa*, the Indian plant being viewed as but an Asiatic condition of that species. . . . The reduction became the more necessary when it was fully understood that, according to climate and soil, the Indian plant varied in as marked a degree as it differed from the European. . . . With *Cannabis indica* differing in so marked a degree according to the climate, soil, and mode of cultivation, it was rightly concluded that its separation from the hemp plant of Europe could not be maintained." Watt compared the hemp plant to potatoes, tobacco, and poppies, all of which "seem to have the power of growing with equal luxuriance under almost any climatic condition, changing or modifying some important function as if to adapt themselves to the altered circumstances."

His opinions were replicated by Dr. D. Prain, who was cited alongside Watt as an expert witness in the commissioners' report. Dr. Prain examined the plant and observed: "There are no botanical characters to separate the Indian plant from *Cannabis sativa*, and they do not differ as regards the structure of stem, leaves, flowers, or fruit. . . . Hemp, therefore, as a fibre-yielding plant in no way differs from hemp as a narcotic-producing one."[20]

The Indian government continued to advocate for the people's right to consume cannabis. When India agreed to prohibit cannabis by signing the United Nations Single Convention on Narcotic Drugs of 1961, it managed to get bhang excluded. Bhang was given another pass when the Parliament of India passed the Narcotic Drugs and Psychotropic Substances Act of 1985 prohibiting the production, sale, transport, and consumption of narcotics, following heavy pressure from the Reagan administration to join the newly invigorated drug war.

Officially and unofficially, cannabis remained available in India, used not only for religious purposes but also as a relaxant and, for many Indians, a means of coping with the hard realities of surviving from day to day. When Harvard physician Lester Grinspoon visited India in 1971, he reported that laborers smoked ganja or drank bhang toward the end of the day because it gave them a sense of well-being, relieved fatigue, stimulated the appetite, and induced a feeling of mild stimulation "which enables the worker to bear more cheerfully the strain of the daily routine of life."[21]

During a pilgrimage to Braj in the early 1990s, religious scholar David L. Haberman encountered many guides who drank bhang daily and religiously. "Drinking or eating bhang prepared in one of a number of delectable forms is said to enhance one's moral qualities and allow deeper emotional experiences," Haberman reported in *Journey through the Twelve Forests: An Encounter with Krishna*. "The state it induces is considered religiously valuable, producing a condition of tranquil yogic insight."[22] The guides told Haberman that bhang was one of four things—along with good food, physical exercise, and singing and meditation on the lord—that contributed to the feeling of being *mast*, or radiant with joy and unburdened by attachments.[23]

In 2009, Richard Connerney wrote in his book, *The Upside-Down Tree: India's Changing Culture*, that customers all across India could walk into state-sanctioned bhang shops, plunk down about $2, and

Bhang and Tantra

In Tibet and Nepal, cannabis became entwined with Tantric yoga, a practice in which consecrated ritualistic sex acts were dedicated to the goddess Kali. About an hour and a half before a couple practicing Tantric sex had intercourse, the devotees uttered several mantras and drank a bowl of bhang. This allowed enough time for the cannabis to take effect so their senses were heightened during the act, expanding their feelings of oneness with Kali.

"buy enough cannabis to induce catatonia for a month." Connerney described a popular drink that could be found all over Benares called a *bhang lassi*, which was basically "hashish mixed with spices and oils." Though he reported dutifully on the thriving, deeply rooted cannabis culture he discovered, Connerney admitted that he was mystified by how the nondescript government bhang stores he encountered could possibly fit within with the "somewhat Byzantine" drug laws in India.[24]

THE MIDDLE EAST: WHERE THE LEGEND OF THE *HASHISHIN* BEGAN

The use of *hashishiyya* (hashish, or concentrated cannabis resin) has a long, rich history in the Middle East, and it is there that much of the pernicious mythology about cannabis's ability to turn men into monsters originated.

As the legend goes, the powers of the cannabis plant were first "discovered" by Sheik Haydar, founder of the Islamic Sufi sect, in 1155. After ten years of solitary meditation, Haydar wandered into the mountains feeling bleak and suicidal, and he came across a trembling cannabis plant. He was drawn to taste its bitter leaves and sticky flowers. When he returned to the monastery a new man, suddenly talkative and full of spirit, his disciples knew they had to learn more about this plant that generated such a striking transformation in their leader. Haydar shared the wealth, saying, "God has granted to you the privilege of knowing the secrets of these leaves. Thus, when you eat it, your dense worries may disappear and your exalted minds become polished. Therefore keep their trust and guard their secrets."

The disciples began to use hashish ritualistically and as an escape from the squalor of having to subsist through begging. They would bathe and change into clean rags before they ate the *luqaynah* ("little morsel"), hash rolled with honey and sesame paste, always touching it only with their right hands.[25] Though luqaynah was most often used as an aid to enhance meditation, Sufis also used it to enhance ecstatic religious states in which they would dance and twirl. Haydar, though he warned his disciples that cannabis could be severely misused in the wrong hands, asked to have cannabis planted around his grave.

In fact, records indicate that hashish was already being widely used in Qumm by the time Haydar "discovered it." Records dating to 1125 tell of Hassan-ibn-Sabbah, also known as the Old Man of the Mountain, a radical missionary heretic and founder of a group of *fedayeen* (people who sacrifice themselves) known as the Assassins. At Eagle's Roost, his isolated castle in Mazandaran mountains near the Caspian Sea, Hassan was said to have given his men majoun as a means of forcing them to perform sinister acts. His misuse of the plant formed the backbone of an epic folk tale that would haunt cannabis for centuries to come.

Hassan, the legend goes, would lure young warriors to a spectacular garden, Shangri-la, where he would provide them with fine food, abundant wine, beautiful virgins, and plenty of majoun made with hashish and opium. Once they were sufficiently drugged and compliant, Hassan would force his disciples to assassinate his political enemies. The inclusion of opium and henbane—much more potent substances—in Hassan's majoun has led to speculation about how much of a role hashish really played in Hassan's sinister manipulation, or original "roofie," but none of that mattered as the legend evolved, over the years, to focus on hashish. The Islamic word for hashish, *hashishin*, is in fact derived from *ashishin*, or assassins.

Many historians believe Persians were the first to sieve dried cannabis flowers to make hashish. In addition to smoking it, they also adopted the practice of making majoun. By the time of the Sassanid Empire (224 to 651 CE), hashish use had spread throughout what would become the Muslim world, used mostly by the lower classes and, therefore, considered a menace to society. *The Thousand and One Nights*, a collection of Middle Eastern folk tales from the Islamic Golden Age, propagated the idea that consuming cannabis led to embarrassment and ridicule through tales of a cannabis-eating fisherman who continuously ended up in embarrassing misadventures. One of the book's stories, "The Tale of the Two Hashish Eaters," described the cartoonish character as "a fisherman by trade and a hashish eater by occupation" who spent his daily wage on a small amount of food and "a sufficiency of that hilarious herb." Because he ate hashish three times a day—in the morning, at noon, and at sundown—"he was never lacking in his extravagant gaiety."[26]

Hashish is said to have fueled the seventh-century prophet Zoroaster as he attempted bridge the gap between heaven and earth while writing *Zend-Avesta*, the Persian counterpart to the Indian Vedas in which Zoroaster described cannabis as a "good narcotic" and said drinking bhang could transport souls to the heavens where the highest mysteries are revealed.[27] In 1123, the first use of the word *hashishiyya* appeared in an official polemic against Isma'ilis, a persecuted Shiite Islami sect.[28] In the twelfth century, Islamic mystics forced by the Mongol invasions to emigrate from Syria to Egypt spread the word about magical majoun as they went, causing a second wave of hashish use.

By the thirteenth century, hashish was sold openly in bazaars and used widely among the lower classes throughout the Muslim world, despite edicts like the one from Sultan Nigm al din Ayoub forbidding people from planting cannabis in the Regouri Gardens and punishing hashish eaters by pulling out their teeth. In writing about his travels in the Middle East, Ibn al-Baytar, an Arab medical herbalist, described encounters with Muslims who were making *hashishah*, also called Indian hemp, and a confection known as a *majoon*, which he said was "very intoxicating," even in small doses. Unlike the sweet, heavily spiced, buttery majoun that the Indians made, the Islamic version was not a confection at all. It was more or less straight hashish, sometimes with a few add-ins. "First, they baked the leaves until they were dry," al-Baytar wrote. "Then, they rubbed them between their hands to form a paste, rolled it into a ball, and swallowed it like a pill. Others dried the leaves only slightly, toasted and husked them, mixed them with sesame and sugar, and chewed them like gum."[29]

Though some historians believe the Crusaders brought the tale of the Old Man of the Mountain and his band of assassins back to Europe as a

Religious Choices

Cultures and religions have been defined—and divided—by their intoxicants of choice throughout history. Early Christians ordained wine and vilified cannabis, despite what many believe to be the Bible's blessing in Genesis 1:29: "Behold, I have given you every herb bearing seed, and to you it will be for meat." Mohammed's followers reached for hashish instead of alcohol, which was forbidden to them.

way of downplaying the bravery of Muslim suicide fighters, it was the Venetian merchant Marco Polo who made the legend known far and wide, through accounts of his journeys through Persia in 1273. Polo's retelling of the tale forever linked hashish with the assassins for most of the world and would be used as fodder for anticannabis propaganda centuries later.

In 1937, when US Federal Bureau of Narcotics chief Harry J. Anslinger was moving full-steam ahead with the "reefer madness" campaign that would force cannabis prohibition in 1937, he called his seminal article "Marihuana: Assassin of Youth" based on the legend of the *hashishin* (a movie was later made with the same name). Anslinger referred to the Old Man of the Mountain when he testified before Congress to launch prohibition, describing the assassins' history of "cruelty, barbarity, and murder" as evidence of how hashish caused people to engage in "violent and bloody deeds."[30]

RUSSIA AND CENTRAL ASIA: CANNABIS "FOR CURE OR PLEASURE"

When the nomadic Scythians began to migrate out from the Caspian Sea to occupy Central Asia and Russia around 3000 BCE, they brought cannabis with them. Medicine Hunter Chris Kilham joked that Scythians invented the first vaporizer based on their legendary tradition of throwing cannabis branches onto heated stones, breathing in the thick, aromatic vapor, and getting really high.

Greek historian Herodotus's description of these rituals would be used again and again by Anslinger and his band of propagandists in their mission to prove that cannabis induced violence and mania. "Scythians put the Seeds of this HEMP under the bags, upon the burning stones; and immediately a more agreeable vapor is emitted than from the incense burnt in Greece," Herodotus wrote. "The Company extremely transported with the scent, howl aloud."[31] (Historians have pointed out that the hot stone ritual was often performed for funerals, which may be a more appropriate reason for the howling.)

In Russia, hemp became known as "Scythian fire" or "Scythian incense," and—as in so many other places around the world—it was popular among the masses and reviled by the upper classes. Hesychius of Alexandria, a lexicographer and grammarian in the fifth and sixth centuries, said hemp had "the power of stealing the youthful vigor of all who stand near." Russian peasants ignored his warnings. Hemp was among the earliest healing plants they used in their folk medicine remedies; a preparation of hemp seeds and flowers to treat toothaches was one of the first to be recorded.

During the Middle Ages, hemp was known in Russia by the Scythian word *penka* and commonly consumed as tea, and beginning in the Czarist Empire of the fifteenth century, and well beyond, Russians celebrated Christmas by offering a soup made from hemp seeds called *semieniata* as food for dead ancestors who were believed to visit on that night.[32]

Hemp seeds and hemp seed oil were staples in Russian and Polish pantries for centuries, and nearly every home, no matter how wealthy its owners, kept a store of them. In a common folk recipe, hemp seeds were bruised and roasted, mixed with salt, and spread onto thick slabs of crusty bread. In Poland, a ubiquitous porridge made from stewed hemp seeds was a subsistence food in monasteries, military barracks, and among the lower classes.[33]

Until the early twentieth century, hemp was an important export for Russia. But when major famines under the Soviets made protein in the form of beef and pork nearly impossible to come by, peasants in Central Russia were forced to live on hemp seed oil as one of their major sources of edible fats. They needed every drop of protein they could get, and all hemp and hemp seed exporting stopped. (By the 1930s, demand for the crop started dropping as the United States pressured the rest of the world to prohibit it along with other narcotics, anyway.)

Russians were also quite fond of smoking and eating hashish for its psychoactive effects, which was highly frowned upon by the Soviets when they took control of Russia in 1922. Citizens of the new regime had to be highly secretive because of the Soviet Union's ongoing efforts to eradicate the hashish trade, but anthropologist Vera Rubin reported finding plenty of people using cannabis, "for cure or pleasure," when she visited the Soviet Union in 1975.

Rubin wrote that Soviets ate, chewed, and smoked cannabis, rubbed it all over their bodies, inhaled it, and made it into elaborate concoctions. She found evidence that people in the Soviet Union used cannabis to successfully cure chronic addiction, particularly alcoholism, in both humans and animals. A common cure for cats who had eaten *mukhomar*, a psychoactive fly agaric mushroom, was to throw them into a cannabis field to let them munch on leaves and flowers until they came to their senses.

Women in Tashkent, Uzbekistan, shared with Rubin their secret recipes, passed down through families for generations, for cannabis-based foods. A traditional favorite was *guc-kand*, a confection made from cannabis, sugar, saffron, and egg whites that parents gave babies to stop them from crying, particularly during circumcision. Women ate *guc-kand* to put themselves in a "happy mood." Another popular dish known as "happy porridge" (or "joy porridge") was made from almond butter mixed with cannabis, dried flower leaves and petals, spices, honey, and sugar. This porridge was very popular among men "who consider it the strongest aphrodisiac," Rubin wrote.[34]

Also revered in Tashkent "as a euphoric agent of pleasure and as a psychoactive aphrodisiac," anthropologist and ethnopharmacologist Christian Rätsch reported in 1998, was a dish made from cannabis and dissolved lamb fat smeared on bread. People also massaged the cannabis-fat mixture into their temples to cure headaches, and women smeared it in their vaginas to lessen the pain of defloration on their wedding nights.[35]

In 2018, *Atlas Obscura* writer Benjamin Kemper set out on a journey through the rough terrain of the Caucasus Mountains in rural Georgia to find and, he hoped, eat a "fragrant, weed-filled iteration" of *khachapuri*, the cheese bread that was a regional staple. The gooey bread was a specialty of the Svans, an ancient community that lived high up in the Caucasus, and all Svans grew cannabis in their gardens until Soviet inspectors arrived and ripped up their plants in the 1990s, a local historian told Kemper. The Svans pressed the seeds for oil and used the flowers, leaves, and ground seeds to make vegetable-walnut spreads (*pkhali*), meat pies (*kubdari*), and cheese breads (*knish*), which were the most important dishes at funerals because of cannabis's association with death.[36]

Kemper's quest was unsuccessful because the Svans had been too afraid to grow cannabis after the Soviet raids of the 1990s, but he may still have a chance. Georgia decriminalized cannabis in late 2017, and the New Centre—the Girchi Party—leader Zurad Japaridze told the *Guardian* he envisioned a number of "weed cafes" opening up in Tbilisi. Those predictions caused speculation that Georgia's largest city could become "the Amsterdam of the former Soviet Union."[37]

EUROPE: HILARITY "WITH OTHER CONFECTIONS"

The Greek historian Herodotus may have made the first mention of cannabis in Western literature in the fifth century BCE when he wrote about the Scythians' howl-inducing vapors, but historians believe Europeans were making use of the plant at least one thousand years before that. Migrating Teutonic tribes, including the Alemannic peoples of the Rhine and Main rivers, are believed to have brought cannabis from the Slavic countries into Germany as early as the second century BCE, and Anglo-Saxon invaders introduced it to the British islands in the fifth century. Storage containers full of cannabis seeds have been found in the remains of Viking ships.[38]

In ancient Europe, pagans and early Christians considered cannabis a magical herb. They used it extensively in religious rituals and incorporated it into their food and medicine. Germanic and Slavic people revered cannabis as a symbol of human and animal fertility, and they found it indispensable as food and medicine. Like every other culture that discovered cannabis before and after them, the pagans made good use of the plant's renowned aphrodisiac powers. In Norway, people consumed cannabis flowers during a festival celebrating Freya, the goddess of love, because they believed the flowers held Freya's feminine, erotic energy, which could be tapped to enhance sexual prowess.

To encourage their growth, early Christian peasants planted cannabis seeds on the days of saints who were known to be tall, such as Saint Christopher. German farmers threw cannabis seeds high into the air and took long strides as they sowed them in a ritual they believed would make the plants more vigorous. In Poland, married women leaped high into the air in a "hemp dance" on Shrove Tuesday, a day of feasting and celebrating before Ash Wednesday. Cannabis spread throughout Europe as a source of food, medicine, and fiber, and it was so important to the economy that many cities had well-established hemp guilds by the late medieval era.

In the fourth century BCE, according to the writings of Greek historian and comedic poet Ephippus, men who gathered to converse and celebrate during gatherings known as *symposia* fueled their conviviality with *kannabides*, confections made from cannabis seeds and honey. Several centuries later, Claudius Galen, Roman emperor Marcus Aurelius's personal physician who promoted a healthy diet based on four "humours" (black bile, yellow bile, blood, and phlegm), wrote about eating small cakes made with cannabis that "increased thirst, but if taken in excess produced torpor (or sluggishness)." Galen wrote that hosts often offered their guests hemp seeds, which they ate to "create warmth" and promote hilarity *cum aliis tragematis* ("with other confections").[39]

The seeds provided far more than nutrition and merriment in Rome, however. Galen also attributed various medicinal qualities to the seeds, all very similar to Ayurvedic medicine's description: "nonflatulent, drying and warming effects, food that harm the head, ability to thin the body's humours and produce 'sticky' and 'cool' humours."[40] In the first century, the physician Dioscorides wrote, Greeks made a popular drink (a basic tincture) by steeping green cannabis seeds in water, wine, or mead for "sufficient days" to extract a liquid known as *khylos*.[41]

Throughout the Middle Ages, cannabis seeds and flowers were put to use in kitchens all across Europe, as evidenced by this recipe for a "health drink of cannabis nectar," a basic extraction found in a cookbook published by papal historian Bartolomeo Platina, the first librarian of the Vatican Library: "Use a mallet to crush clods collected after a good harvest. Add cannabis to nard oil in an iron pot, crush together over some heat and liquefy." Platina included a warning about the beverage's psychoactive potency and some sage advice as well. "Carefully treat food and divide for the stomach and the head," he wrote. "Finally, remember everything in excess may be harmful or criminal."[42]

Indeed, by the late fifteenth century, disapproval from the Vatican effectively stopped all use of cannabis as an intoxicant in Europe, except for the very underground, until the late eighteenth century, when Napoleon's troops brought hashish back from their invasions in Egypt[43] and the book *One Thousand and One Nights*, with many references to hashish, was widely circulated in Europe. Napoleon also tried to outlaw all cannabis use, but it was too late. The glories of eating hashish had been revealed to the European intelligentsia, and it would soon be all the rage among the literati.

• 3 •

Revelry and Revilement

In the 1830s, Jacques-Joseph Moreau, a renowned pioneering French psychiatrist who was the first doctor to systematically study the effect of drugs on the central nervous system, discovered hashish during his travels through the Middle East and began to explore the legend of Hassan-ibn-Sabbah, the Old Man of the Mountain, and his band of assassins. In his 1845 book *Hashish and Mental Illness*, Moreau—the first psychiatrist to suggest that cannabis could be a useful tool in treating psychosis—hypothesized that the psychoactive effects of cannabis might be similar to the hallucinations and delusions that people have with psychosis.

Moreau believed that all mental health professionals and researchers should imbibe hashish because experiencing psychotic symptoms themselves would allow them to better understand their patients. His book outlined the process hashish users go through as they progressively lose control of their faculties and emotions through eight stages, from an initial feeling of pure happiness to "development of the sense of hearing" in stage four, when "the crudest music, the simplest vibrations of the strings of a harp or a guitar, rouse you to a point of delirium or plunge you into a sweet melancholy."[1] This "manic excitement," Moreau wrote, was always accompanied by "a feeling of gaiety and joy inconceivable to those who have never experienced it. I saw in it a means of effectively combatting the fixed ideas of depressives, disrupting the chain of their ideas, of unfocusing their attention on such and such a subject."[2]

While Moreau was in Algiers, he learned how to make *dawamesk*, a variation of majoun made from hashish, sugar, vanilla, almonds, musk, pistachio, cinnamon, orange extract, cloves, cardamom, nutmeg, and often a small amount of cantharides (Spanish fly), a beetle secretion believed to be an aphrodisiac that would have "greatly raised the potential for serious damage to the user, since the lethal dose of cantharides is relatively low and varies greatly from person to person," Lester Grinspoon wrote in *Marihuana Reconsidered*.[3] Moreau was immediately hooked on the confection's psychoactive pleasures and eager to share the "little green sweetmeat" while reenacting the dramatic antics of his hero, the Old Man of the Mountain.

He invited his friend, the outspoken hedonist and popular novelist Théophile Gautier, to partake in a dinner in which Moreau would ritualistically feed diners dawamesk so he could record their reactions. Gautier, never one to turn down a party, recruited a few fellow literati, including poet and essayist Charles Baudelaire, author and playwright Alexandre Dumas, novelist and dramatist Victor Hugo, novelist and playwright Honoré de Balzac, and painter Eugene Delacroix, to join the party. *Le Club des Hachichins*—the not-so-secret society that would introduce millions of Westerners to the joys and perils of eating hashish—was born.

The club members met once a month from 1844 until 1849 at the grand, gothic Hotel Pimodan in Paris for a ritual based on the legend of Hassan and his assassins. Moreau, often dressed in a traditional Turkish costume of a loose coat over baggy trousers, dispensed the hashish confection from a crystal bowl as he told each member, "This will be deducted from your share in paradise." The doctor didn't partake himself, but he recorded in detail what happened to his fellow members. Other members reported firsthand accounts, in even more lurid detail, of their extremely intense journeys at the Hotel Pimodan, which both intrigued and alarmed the reading classes.

In his article "*Le Club des Hachichins*," published in the *Revue des Deux Mondes* in 1846, Gautier gave up a full description of his night with the no-longer-clandestine club. He described Moreau, his face radiant with enthusiasm, eyes glittering, purple cheeks aglow, veins popping out in his temples, and breathing heavily through dilated nostrils as he handed Gautier his portion of the sweet, green paste. The effects of the hallucinogenic appetizer began to come on during the elaborate banquet, Gautier wrote. "Water . . . seemed to savor like the most delicate wine, the meat turned to raspberries in my mouth, and conversely, I could not have told a cutlet from a peach."

The faces of the diners around him changed shape and color as some became agitated, some laughed hilariously, and some struggled to raise their glasses. After dinner, while listening to "celestial choirs," Gautier found everything "larger, richer, more gorgeous" as he enjoyed "the splendors of the hallucination." The drawing room filled with weird beings and shapes, "coming together with sad looks and shaking hands with a melancholy cordiality, like persons afflicted with a common sorrow. They were saying: 'Time is dead. Henceforth, there will be no years, no months, no hours; time is dead, and we are going to its funeral.'"

Gautier also experienced a state that is known as synesthesia in which the senses are mixed up so that people "smell" colors and "see" sounds and feelings. "The notes quivered with such power that they entered my breast like luminous arrows . . . sounds sprang forth, blue and red, in electric sparks," he wrote.[4]

In analyzing Gautier's accounts, Grinspoon noted that it was important to consider "set and setting," the physical, mental, and social context and environment that would have influenced Gautier's hashish experiences. Grinspoon pointed out that Gautier's psychological "set" was apparently one of extreme nervous expectation, and the general "setting," a formal dining room in the baroque Hotel Pimodan where the club met, was "at the very least macabre."

The club members reportedly took massive doses of hashish, and their experiences were not something many people could or would want to replicate. "The effusive descriptions of such writers as Gautier, Taylor, Baudelaire, and Ludlow are, however, often excessive and distorted and frequently have little to do with the moderate use of cannabis (e.g., the smoking of marihuana)," Grinspoon wrote, "for they were written about and under the influence of large amounts of ingested hashish, sometimes admixed with other drugs."[5]

Many historians believe that in addition to Spanish fly, the dawamesk that Moreau fed the club members also contained opium, which could have contributed to or even been responsible for Gautier's and others' severe reactions. Baudelaire, who often criticized hashish and only very rarely partook in the dawamesk during the club's dinners, affirmed this in his essay, "On Wine and Hashish," published in a book he cowrote with Gautier, *Hashish, Wine, Opium.* Baudelaire described hashish as "composed of a decoction of Indian hemp, butter, and a small quantity of opium"[6] and also confirmed that Spanish fly was included in the confection.

For Baudelaire, the Spanish fly was a welcome addition because he believed it softened the effects of the other substances. "Under this new form hashish has no disagreeable qualities, and one can take it in a dose of fifteen, twenty, and thirty grammes, either enveloped in a leaf of pain a chanter or in a cup of coffee," Baudelaire wrote in "The Poem of Hashish," published in his 1860 book *Le Paradis Artificiels* (*Artificial Paradise*). He added that hashish's effects could vary extremely, "according to the individual temperament and nervous susceptibility of the hashish-eater."[7] And Baudelaire also reported experiencing synesthesia. "Sounds take on colours, and colours contain music," he wrote.

Gautier's and Baudelaire's essays introduced French intelligentsia to hashish, but it was Dumas's eloquent descriptions of the euphoria that eating hash induced, in his 1844 book *The Count of Monte Cristo*, that piqued the interest of readers throughout Europe. In the wildly popular adventure tale, hashish played a predominant role as an aphrodisiac and sedative with the ability to produce pleasant dreams and indescribable well-being.

Dumas wrote that eating hashish could enhance people's experience of music to the point where they could hear the "seven choirs of paradise." In one chapter of *The Count of Monte Cristo*, a man who called himself Sinbad the Sailor invited a young Frenchman named Franz d'Epinay to dine with him in his sumptuously decorated cave on the island of Monte Cristo, and Franz told his host to call him Aladdin because the evening felt like an *Arabian Nights* adventure. After dinner, a Nubian servant brought two baskets filled with desserts and a small, silver cup with a silver cover that he placed with great care between the baskets. His curiosity aroused, Franz lifted the lid and saw "a greenish paste, something like preserved angelica, but which was perfectly unknown to him."

In his explanation about the "sweetmeat," Sinbad recounted Marco Polo's tale about the Old Man of the Mountain, and he invited the young man to try it. Franz ate a teaspoon full of the jam and floated away on a beautiful trip.

> His body seemed to acquire an airy lightness, his perception brightened in a remarkable manner, his senses seemed to redouble their

> power, the horizon continued to expand; but it was not the gloomy horizon of vague alarms, and which he had seen before he slept, but a blue, transparent, unbounded horizon, with all the blue of the ocean, all the spangles of the sun, all the perfumes of the summer breeze; then, in the midst of the songs of his sailors—songs so clear and sonorous, that they would have made a divine harmony had their notes been taken down—he saw the Island of Monte Cristo, no longer as a threatening rock in the midst of the waves, but as an oasis in the desert.[8]

AMERICAN HASH EATERS: "PRODIGIOUS APPARENT ENLARGEMENT OF THE BRAIN"

Just as *The Count of Monte Cristo* and other works by the *hashishin* club members were inspiring hashish mania in Europe, American travel writer Bayard Taylor published *The Land of the Saracens*, a book in which he described his experiences after eating a large dose—six times as much as most people ate—of "hasheesh" while he was traveling in Egypt. Bayard described eating a paste, "made from the leaves of the plant, mixed with sugar and spices" that tasted "aromatic and slightly pungent, but by no means disagreeable," and then "paying a frightful penalty for my curiosity." His majoun trip plunged him into a hellish nightmare that lasted for hours.

"Yet, fearful as my rash experiment proved to me, I did not regret having made it," Taylor wrote. "It revealed to me deeps of rapture and of suffering which my natural faculties never could have sounded. It has taught me the majesty of human reason and of human will, even in the weakest, and the awful peril of tampering with that which assails their integrity." Taylor, well aware that a good number of curiosity seekers like himself would have to have a taste of the exotic confection, even after hearing about the horrors he experienced, beseeched his readers to "take the portion of hasheesh which is considered sufficient for one man, and not, like me, swallow enough for six."[9]

That was all the encouragement American writer Fitz Hugh Ludlow needed. A cultishly popular autobiographical author, whom ethnobotanist Terence McKenna described as "a kind of Mark Twain on hashish" and credited with launching "a tradition of pharmo-picaresque literature that would find later practitioners in William Burroughs and Hunter S. Thompson," Ludlow ran to the pharmacy and got his hands on a hash-based medicine called Tilden's Cannabis Indica as soon as he finished reading *The Land of the Saracens.*

Ludlow completely ignored Taylor's advice and experimented with extremely high doses of the hashish elixir. He recorded his experiences, as well as his philosophies about religion, medicine, and culture, in his 1857 book *The Hasheesh Eater: Being Passages from the Life of a Pythagorean*, which would become required literature for the Beats and hippies a century later.

Ludlow wrote that when he was under the influence of hashish, "objects which appear to ordinary, utilitarian, pragmatic, goal-oriented thought and perception as irrelevant take on sudden and surprisingly fresh meanings." He described hashish intoxication as "the sudden nervous thrill, followed by the whirl and prodigious apparent enlargement of the brain. My head expanded wider and wider, revolving with inconceivable rapidity, and enlarging in space with every revolution."[10] Published by Harper and Brothers, one of the nation's most prestigious presses, *The Hasheesh Eater* was a runaway success and launched the first national conversation about cannabis in the United States.

Hashish became the darling of the New York literati—and soon moved well beyond those elite circles and into the mainstream. At the 1877 World's Fair Centennial Exposition in Philadelphia, an international spectacle where representatives from all over the world scrambled to outdo each other with exotic exhibits and unveiled exciting new inventions such as the telephone, people stood in long lines to get a taste of hashish from a long pipe known as a hookah at the Turkish Pavilion, and some enthusiasts took smoking devices home with them as "souvenirs." After the fair, Turkish smoking parlors began cropping up in every major city from New York to Chicago. Manhattan and San Francisco became overrun with them, sounding the alarm for the press and leading to an eventual crackdown.

In a sensationalized and largely inaccurate article titled "The Secret Dissipation of New York Belles . . . a Hasheesh Hell on Fifth Avenue," the *Illustrated Police News* described these "tea pads" as luxurious private clubs where "young dandies" smoked and ate hashish. *Harper's Monthly* described a very different kind of scene in its article "A Hashish-House in New York," published in 1883.[11] The author, H. H. Kane, visited a house where women and men of "the better classes" went to eat "*majoon*," small, black lozenges made from cannabis resin, butter, sugar, honey, flour, henbane, crushed datura seeds, and opium. Tea made from coca leaves was also available. Kane partook of the majoon and prepared to be transported to a state that his host described as "hashishdom," a sense of "perfect rest and strange, quiet happiness" that had been drawing a growing number of habitués to tea houses for the past two years.

Kane was not so lucky. Instead of floating away on pink clouds, he was vaulted into a hellish hallucination involving a large-nosed "chemist of the earth's bowels" who played "a harmony, a symphony, of odors" on a huge, curiously constructed organ as well as a committee of frightening spirits, "still incarnate, of individuals who, during life, sought happiness in the various narcotics." Kane eventually managed to escape the tea house, but he couldn't escape the spirits. They clung to him, their scrawny arms wound about his neck, in his hair, on his limbs, "pulling me over into the horrible chasm, into the heart of hell."

With nothing else to do, Kane walked through the streets of New York in a drizzling rain until the majoun began to wear off. As it did, he began to deeply appreciate everything around him—the odors, sounds, and sights of "the cradle of dreams rocking placidly in the very heart of a great city, translated from Baghdad to Gotham."[12]

JAMAICA: "DE HEALIN' OF DE NATION"

There is perhaps no other country in the world where cannabis plays such a major role in the economy and in people's social and spiritual lives as in Jamaica.

Ganja, as it is known on the island, was introduced to Jamaican sugar plantation workers by indentured servants from India who were imported by the British authorities to help work the fields after slavery was abolished in 1834. The Indian workers brought ganja seeds as well as a deep-seated cultural affinity for smoking it in *chillums*, and they built a thriving cottage industry growing and selling ganja and smoking paraphernalia among themselves. Once the former slaves who worked alongside them discovered the herb's ability to ease the pain of their brutal working conditions and extreme poverty, they began saving seeds and planting their own gardens.

Much like the colonialists who ruled India, the plantation owners in Jamaica tolerated workers' use of ganja, as well as the island's other favorite intoxicant, rum, because it kept the laborers pacified and able to maintain the merciless pace of harvesting sugar under a baking sun in the hot, humid fields or turning it into rum in the sweltering, grindingly dangerous mills and factories—for twelve hours a day or more. In Trenchtown, a massive ghetto of cardboard shacks that was built up over a sewage trench on the outskirts of Kingston as more and more Jamaicans sought to escape hopeless conditions in rural areas, ganja was a key thread in the community fabric, perhaps the only means for most people to escape the grueling destitution of their daily lives.

Throughout the island, cannabis was bought and sold openly, available even in company stores, until rum production and exporting surged in the early twentieth century. With economies of scale, manufacturers were able to drastically drop the price of rum, making it competitive with ganja—and British colonialists knew how to compete. Missionaries and government officials began a massive public relations campaign against ganja, which they called the "vile weed." Their crusades, a brutal type of class and race warfare, resulted in cannabis being declared illegal in 1913.

Criminalization, which brought persecution and dire consequences to Jamaicans caught using ganja, was a masterful way of keeping workers oppressed, but it did nothing to stop the island's thriving cannabis economy and culture. "Outlawing a popular custom is also a very convenient control device," Dr. Lambros Comitas, who with Vera D. Rubin visited Jamaica to conduct one of the most comprehensive anthropological studies of the island that had ever been undertaken in the 1970s, explained to *High Times*. "The ganja legislation in Jamaica is very clearly like the legislation against illegitimate children or against obeah, a particular form of lower-class religion. It can be used by the elite to control the lower classes with no loss in world opinion."[13]

In 1932, Leonard Percival Howell, a charismatic Jamaican preacher who had been running one of the many tea houses that had opened up in New York's Harlem, was deported. Howell returned to his homeland, where his black-liberation sermons inspired by the

Bible and Jamaican black nationalist Marcus Garvey began to draw ever-increasing crowds all across the island. Howell told Jamaicans that the first black African leader, Ras Tafari Makonnen, Emperor Haile Selassie I of Ethiopia, was messiah returned to earth. Followers of Howell's philosophy became known as Rastafarians, and the movement grew into a religion (though it would never be recognized as such by law).

Citing Psalms 104:14—"He causeth the grass to grow for the cattle, and herb for the service of man, that he may bring forth food out of the earth"—Rastafarians considered ganja a holy herb and used it as part of their religious and sacramental rites. They believed God, or Jah, revealed himself through herbs—primarily ganja—that were put on earth to solve the rifts between people of different nations and help people connect with Jah. In one of his most frequently repeated quotes, reggae superstar and world's most famous Trenchtown Rasta, Bob Marley, told the *New York Times* in 1977: "Herb is a natural ting, It grow like de tree. It is de healin' of de nation. I cannot use it jus to get high. Me no do dat. De herb inspires. It clears ya out."[14]

Rastafarianism took hold of Jamaica and became a key part of the island's culture and governance, especially after the country gained independence from the United Kingdom in 1962.

A 1966 visit from Emperor Haile Selassie himself drew enthusiastic throngs of Rastafarian elders as well as new converts. Six years later, People's National Party leader Michael Manley drove audiences at his political rallies wild when he waved his "rod of correction," which Selassie had given him, during his "Better Must Come" campaign in 1972. Manley, the first Jamaican politician to support the Rastafarians, won the election and became one of the nation's most popular prime ministers ever during his rule from 1972 to 1980.

Under Manley, Rastafarianism continued to thrive, showing no signs of retreat, even after Selassie's death in 1975. A good six out of ten Jamaicans were Rastafarians,[15] and the *New York Times* reported in 1976 that Rastafarians had been "the prevailing cultural force in Jamaica for thirty years and are the major influence over young Jamaicans today."[16] Manley's move to lower the minimum voting age in Jamaica to eighteen made that influence even greater, as young voters helped elect Rastafarians to government positions and elders took on authority roles within greater communities.

Manley implemented a series of reforms designed to address the severely skewed wealth distribution that had plagued Jamaica since colonialism and slavery—hence his "We Can Do Better" campaign—with mixed results. The reforms were not enough to seriously affect the crippling poverty and chronic unemployment in large rural swatches as well as the urban slums. Manley's land-lease program, however, was a crucial development for Rastafarians, and their ability to grow ganja in particular. By leasing land to small farmers for five-year periods, the program paved the way for Rastafarian communities to become self-sufficient and carry out their spiritual beliefs, which included cultivating their own fruits, vegetables, and herbs. "Like ganja," they said, "the earth brings forth all good things."[17]

The program brought a measure of hope to rural Jamaicans and led to thriving agricultural ganja-growing collectives such as Orange Hill in Negril and Nine Mile in the central mountains, where Bob Marley lived. Still, ganja remained illegal, if widely tolerated. Farmers were forced to work through underground channels, without protection, knowing they could be oppressed for their efforts or have their crops eradicated at any moment—by their own government or the United States.

In June 1974, claiming it was working at the request of the Jamaican government, the US DEA launched its first major paramilitary action abroad in the war against cannabis on the island. The DEA's all-out assault, engineered to eradicate the crop that was increasingly making its way to the eastern shores of the United States, involved aircraft, helicopters, flamethrowers, and herbicides, and it scorched a full one-fifth of Jamaica's ground surface. The purpose, according to *High Times*, was to "destroy the island's third-largest industry and intimidate the 70 percent of the population who support it."[18]

Among the poverty-ridden—most of the island's population—ganja use was extensive. In 1975, when anthropologists Comitas and Rubin visited Jamaica, they reported that ganja use was "extraordinarily widespread," estimating the number of users ranged from one-third to two-thirds of the "lower class"—nearly the entire nation considering that 5 percent of the island's residents owned 95 percent of its wealth.

At least 25 percent of all Jamaican households included someone who cultivated cannabis, with harvests in August and November, the anthropologists found. Jamaicans smoked it, used it in teas and tonics believed to strengthen the blood and ward off disease, and used it extensively in the kitchen, stirring it into soups, tossing it with assorted greens, and eating it with cooked bananas.[19]

Cannabis was used liberally in the Rastafarian *ital* diet, which rejects artificial and processed food, meat, sugar, dairy, and alcohol—all of which Rastafarians consider detrimental effects of consumerist society, or what they call Babylon—in favor of fresh fruits, vegetables, and herbs. Ital dishes, often one-pot stews cooked over open coals, are made using local produce such as yams, peppers, onions, a beloved local green called *callaloo*, scotch bonnet, and allspice. The word *ital* is derived from the word *vital*, meaning "essential to life," and the diet is based on the Bible's edict that the body is a temple and must be kept clean. Rastafarians believe the ital way of eating creates *livity*, universal energy or life force.

Eating live, raw, uncooked food was the right thing to do because that's how Adam and Eve ate, Rastafari leader Ras Iyah V told Harvard University Law School professor Charles Nesson during a 2017 interview in which he described the lifestyle he had led for the past forty-two years. "Before fire, holy man live, holy man eat," he said. "Where I'm from, in Jamaica, we have a lot of fruits, a lot of vegetables. From an Edenic point of view, people naturally eat what home and nature could provide before they made fire."

Not only that, Ras Iyah said, but eating fruits and vegetables in their raw state was the only way to absorb all of their nutritional and health benefits. "I learned in school, in chemistry, that heat will destroy enzymes," he said. "When the enzymes are gone out of your food, the metabolic and digestion process tends to become more difficult. That's why I choose not to eat cooked food."[20]

Not all cannabis-laced food in Jamaica was so healthy. Enterprising bakers began selling ganja-laced brownies and cakes on Jamaica's beaches to a new market of tourists who were hungry for pot brownies after discovering them at home in the late 1960s. By the late 1970s and 1980s, hipper travel guides and even conservative entities like the *Chicago Tribune* were sending Jamaican tourists in search of cannabis-infused treats (as well as tea brewed from psilocybin mushrooms, which were never illegal in Jamaica) to Jenny's Famous Cakes and Miss Brown's Fine Foods in Negril—a place that was already legendary when ethnobotanist Chris Kilham bought a cake there and, in his words, "tripped my face off for thirteen hours" in 1988.

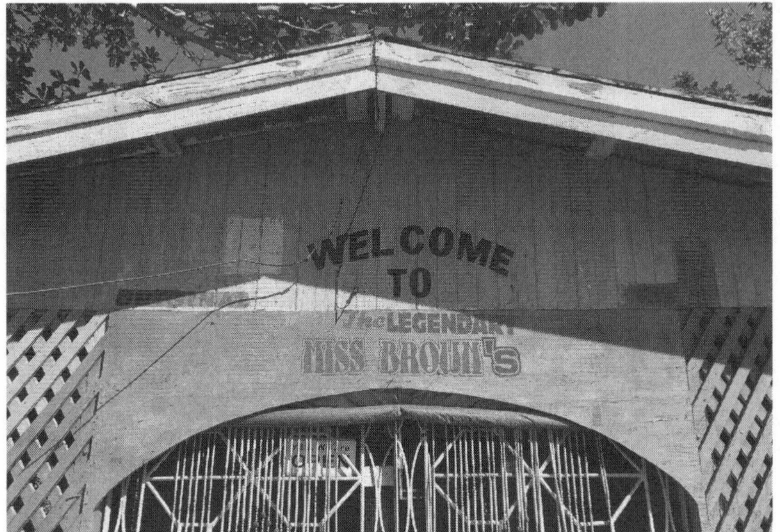

Miss Brown's has been serving cannabis-infused brownies and cakes in Negril, Jamaica, since the 1980s. Photo by Chris Kilham.

Miss Brown's continued to sell brownies, cakes, and tea for more than two decades, but it had fallen into disrepair—"like an abandoned amusement," Kilham said—when he returned to Negril in 2017 and immediately made a pilgrimage to the small shack he remembered fondly (see photo above). Kilham said the $15 slice of dense chocolate cake he bought tasted too obviously of hash oil. "It just didn't have the same charm. Frankly, I didn't enjoy the flavor," he said. "In terms of intensity, there's no question Miss Brown's is upholding its bargain as the stratospheric space cake on the island. But qualitatively, it was kind of sad."

Kilham visited two years after the Jamaican government made the game-changing move of decriminalizing cannabis, legalizing medical marijuana, and making it legal for Jamaicans to grow five plants per household in 2015. Qualified medical marijuana patients from anywhere in the world could buy and use cannabis in Jamaica, and possession of less than two ounces garnered tourists and locals a ticket instead of a jail sentence and a criminal record.

The governmental change of heart about a crop once vilified and used as a means of persecuting Rastafarians came as Jamaicans watched other places like Colorado rake in millions after legalizing the plant Jamaica had come to be renowned for all over the world. The Jamaican government saw cannabis as a key component in lifting the country out of its dismal economic growth rate, one of the lowest in the developing world, and announced plans to create a global hub for medical cannabis research and cannabis-centered health and wellness tourism. "Jamaica for so long has been associated with this plant," Doug Gordon, who organized the first CanEx conference for government and local leaders to talk about the new industry in 2016, told the *New York Times*. "Now, it's a business, an opportunity, one that can change the future of this country through jobs and income, one that can change our GDP."

Ras Iyah V, who served as chairman of the Westmoreland Hemp and Ganja Farmers Association and was an executive member of the Cannabis Licensing Authority, which was created in 2015 to establish and regulate Jamaica's newly legal cannabis industry, told the *Jamaica Gleaner* in 2017 that he believed Jamaica's political leaders had allowed the United States to "dictate Jamaica's drug policy, resulting in the destruction of our *ganja* supply" while at the same time ensuring that a flourishing cannabis industry could get underway at home.

The Rastafarian elder was pleased about the new laws, but he also told the newspaper he did not support the manufacture and sale of cannabis-infused edibles, which were extremely popular in states that had legalized in the United States. "Reason being," he said, "most of the individuals who provide these products have little to no scientific knowledge about ganja."[21]

The first legal cannabis plant was put in Jamaican ground at the University of the West Indies Mona campus in April 2015, and the first legal medical marijuana dispensary, Kaya Herb House, opened in Ocho Rios with much fanfare and a concert featuring longtime reggae favorites Toots and the Maytals in 2018.

In Negril, in 2017, there was a giddiness. Everyone from cab drivers to business owners to cannabis growers talked about the difference decriminalization made for them. Locals could no longer lose their right to ever leave the island again over a possession charge. Roadside extortion and crop eradication became things of the past.

Though ganja wasn't technically legal, plenty of enterprising people began to treat it that way in those early years after it was decriminalized in 2015. Entrepreneurs built businesses first and asked permission second, largely because the licensing fees required under the new laws were out of reach for small farmers and businesses. "They want $2,500 American," said the owner of a café that sold cannabis-infused smoothies, muffins, popcorn, and other treats from two bright, well-maintained shacks on the beach and up in the cliffs in Negril. "Do you know how many brownies I would have to sell to make that?"

At the 2017 Rastafari Rootzfest, a government-sanctioned annual reggae festival and ganja market held in December on Long Beach in Negril, vendors sold homemade cannabis-infused brownies, gummies, cakes, muffins, and pieces of pie swathed in cling wrap alongside booths offering huge bouquets of cannabis branches and massive balls of hash (see photo below). The crowd, made up mostly of dreadlocked Rastafarians wearing the red, green, and black colors of their religion, was jubilant.

During a rousing speech, Balram Vaswani, who saw a nearly twenty-year-old dream come true when he opened Jamaica's first medi-

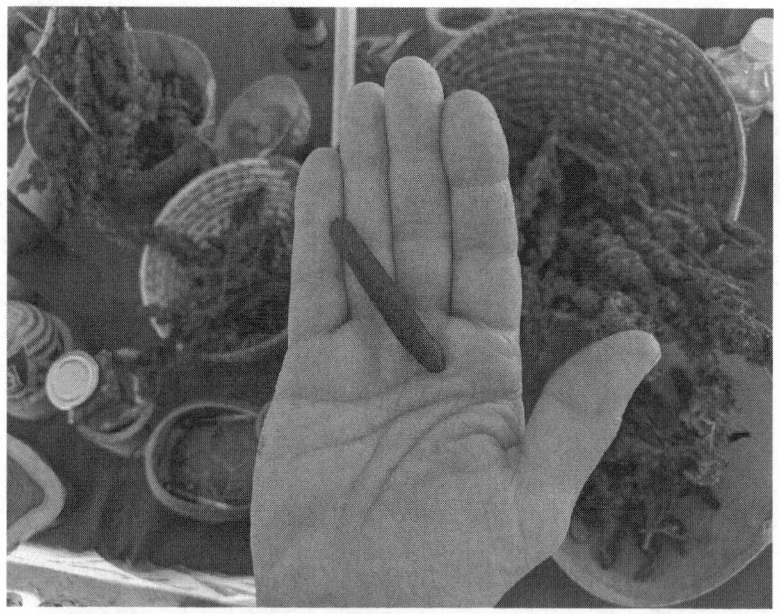

A finger of hashish for sale at the Rastafari Rootzfest in Negril, Jamaica. Photo by Zoe Helene.

cal marijuana dispensary, Kaya Herb House, in 2018, told festival goers that Jamaica had been the victim of cash grabs by foreigners in everything from sugar to coffee to tourism, but said that would not happen with cannabis. "We're smart enough now," he said, "to prevent that exploitation."

THE UNITED STATES: DECADES OF REEFER MADNESS

In the mid-nineteenth century, Dr. W. B. O'Shaughnessy's reports from India's Bengal province about the promise of cannabis as a treatment for a range of illnesses began to reach America. The American medical community, intrigued by the possibility of cures that had eluded Western doctors, embraced cannabis and began to prescribe it as medicine. *C. sativa* and *C. indica* became common ingredients in readily available over-the-counter elixirs and tinctures until well into the twentieth century.

Americans swallowed cannabis in these tinctures at daily dosages "equal to what a current moderate-to-heavy American marijuana user probably consumes in a month or two," legendary cannabis advocate Jack Herer reported in his procannabis classic *The Emperor Wears No Clothes*, and they were Americans' favorite type of medicine for decades. The authors of marriage guides in the 1890s recommended cannabis as a potent aphrodisiac, and temperance organizations suggested hashish as a substitute for alcohol. But when the invention of the hypodermic syringe made heroin easier to administer, Herer wrote, doctors stopped using cannabis because it was difficult to standardize the dosing and they couldn't shoot up patients with it using their "new injectable needle."[22]

Though cannabis tinctures were not as popular as the new pharmaceuticals that began to emerge in the late nineteenth century, cannabis-based medicines remained available and unremarkable until the 1930s, when the US government unleashed an all-out global war against cannabis that would reverberate throughout the world for the next century. Following a brilliantly executed propaganda campaign and global arm-twisting led by US Federal Bureau of Narcotics director

Harry J. Anslinger, the elixirs Americans relied on to ease their daily aches and pains were made illegal, alongside the dried cannabis flowers that Mexican immigrants and jazz musicians enjoyed smoking, and industrial hemp, which the popular press—not understanding its connection to the evil narcotic they were vilifying—was at the same time heralding as the crop of the future.

The seeds of Anslinger's war were actually planted long before Anslinger, south of the border in Mexico. In 1896, the Associated Press–associated English-language newspaper the *Mexican Herald* reported that much of the *pulque*, a viscous, milk-colored drink made from fermented maguey (agave) that was sold in Mexico City markets, was adulterated with "marihuana," a drug that caused "temporary madness" and caused people to "pull out knives and stab their comrades upon the slightest provocation." The authors of this article had cannabis confused with the hallucinogenic nightshade plant *Datura stramonium*, known on the street as jimsonweed, but that didn't matter to the hundreds of newspapers and magazines that picked up the story off the wire and ran it under blaring and sensational headlines in the United States.[23]

As Mexico became engulfed in violence and chaos during the years leading up to the Mexican Revolution in 1910, politicians and yellow journalists sought out topics that would direct citizens' ire elsewhere, and cannabis was an easy target. They launched a propaganda campaign that reached so far and so wide that apparently even largely illiterate lower-class Mexicans were well aware of the plant's evils. One commentator reported in 1908: "The horror that this plant inspires has reached such an extreme that when the common people see even just a single plant, they feel as if in the presence of a demonic spirit. Women and children run frightened, and they make the sign of the cross simply upon hearing its name."[24] The Mexican government labeled marijuana a threat that could "degenerate the race" and banned it nationwide in 1920.[25]

The Mexican Revolution sent thousands of Mexicans fleeing up north to the United States, and many of them—unconvinced by the propaganda campaign from a government they distrusted—brought with them their longtime practice of rolling up dried cannabis flowers and smoking them and sometimes mixing cannabis into tea, coffee, or *pulque*. The anticannabis scare campaign followed the immigrants across the border, and soon journalists in the United States were pumping out articles about a frightening new drug called *marijuana*. (The spelling of the word, which is Mexican slang for "intoxicate," changed from the original *h* to a *j* in American newspapers starting around 1910, and many people argue that the propagandists did that to make the plant seem more foreign and frightening.) The word *marijuana* entered the general lexicon on both sides of the border through the lyrics of "La Cucaracha," a marching song adopted by Pancho Villa's troops, who were said to use cannabis to keep themselves alert and amused during long cavalry rides.

Brought by Mexican immigrants and sailors from the Caribbean islands to New Orleans, cannabis smoking was picked up by jazz musicians, who made no secret of their love for the herb in songs referring to it as muggles, *mota*, gage, tea, reefer, Mary Warner, Mary Jane, and *rosa maria*. Cab Calloway praised the gage in "The Reefer Man," and Louis Armstrong, who called cannabis "a friend" and said it was "a thousand times better than alcohol," tooted its horn in "Muggles." Fats Waller sang "got to get high before I sing" in "Viper's Drag," and Bessie Smith sang, "give me a reefer and a gang of gin." Even Benny Goodman serenaded the gage in "Texas Tea Party" and "Sweet Marihuana Brown."

The streets of New Orleans' largely black Storyville neighborhood, where Armstrong—and jazz—were born, were packed with tea pads where, to the horror of city officials, black and white people danced together and shared cannabis. In 1910, the New Orleans Public Safety Commissioner wrote that there were more than two hundred users of marijuana, "the most frightening and vicious drug ever to hit New Orleans," in Storyville alone. "Marijuana's insidious evil influence apparently manifested itself in making the 'darkies' think they were as good as 'white men,'" wrote Herer, who couldn't escape the irony that "American newspapers, politicians, and police had virtually no idea until the 1920s, and then only rarely, that the marijuana the 'darkies' and 'Chicanos' were smoking in cigarettes or pipes was just a weaker version of the many familiar cannabis medicines they'd been taking since childhood or the weaker drug of the local 'white man's' plush hashish parlors."[26]

Musicians and migrant workers carried cannabis up the Mississippi River to urban centers in the north, where tea pads blossomed. The new trend, popular among bohemians and people of color, inevitably caught the attention of the federal government. In 1906, egged on by the increasingly powerful new pharmaceutical industry, the US government enacted the Pure Food and Drug Act, which established truth-in-labeling requirements for food and medicine. The strict requirements spelled the end of nearly all of the patent medicines available over the counter to American consumers, who increasingly turned to prescription drugs, and was the first nail in the coffin for cannabis in the United States.

In another development that many believe was the kiss of death for cannabis in America, the decorticator, invented by George Schlichten in 1917, dramatically reduced the labor required to separate hemp fibers from the stalks. This marvelous new invention brought the cost of making hemp paper down to about half the cost of making paper from trees. That got the attention of powerful industrialist William Randolph Hearst, who saw cheaper, more efficient hemp production as a threat to his timberland empire. Some say Hearst also held a grudge against all Mexicans after Pancho Villa's army seized 800,000 acres of his timberland in Mexico.

For whatever reason, Hearst used his newspaper empire to link the "scary" Mexican drug marijuana to sensational acts of torture and murder. Hearst's journalists wrote hundreds of articles positioning marijuana as an evil drug used by seductive, dark-haired "senoritas" to turn young people into violent lunatics and by dark-skinned, satanic-looking men to have their way with young white women. The flurry of articles created, according to cannabis historian Barney J. Warf, a moral panic "conveniently fed by the potential competition that hemp offered to producers of paper, textiles, and synthetic fiber"[27]—and a healthy dose of racism. In a recent interview, Warf explained: "Nothing gets good WASP morals aflame more than the idea that evil men were using cannabis to seduce women. In particular, black men doing it to white women. That's a mainstay of white racist discourses and hyperbole."[28]

Article after article told of women who smoked marijuana and then slept with black men and violent Mexican immigrants who were emboldened to carry out atrocious acts after using the drug, and the pervasive narrative terrified white people in the deeply racist United States. State governments, starting with California and Utah, sprang to action, passing laws that outlawed marijuana throughout the 1910s and 1920s. When the Colorado legislature outlawed cannabis in 1917, it stated that Mexicans under marijuana's influence were "demanding humane treatment, looking at white women, and asking that their children be educated while the parents harvest sugar beets, and other 'insouciant' demands."[29]

The United States' anticannabis crusade, already rolling quite along, took on a life of its own in 1930, when Treasury Secretary Andrew Mellon appointed Anslinger, his future nephew-in-law, to be head of the new Federal Bureau of Narcotics and Dangerous Drugs, tasked with stamping out cannabis along with narcotics such as heroin and cocaine in the United States. Some historians conjecture that, at the same time, Mellon gave Anslinger a portfolio of stocks in companies that were developing products that competed with hemp, such as Gulf Oil, so the new drug czar would have his own financial stake in stamping out cannabis.

Anslinger went after cannabis with a vengeance, feeding a hungry cadre of journalists—not all of them yellow—who were all too happy to take his bait. In 1934, the venerable *New York Times* published an article with a series of alarming headlines: "Use of Marijuana Spreading in West, Poisonous Weed Is Being Sold Quite Freely in Pool Halls and Beer Gardens. Children Said to Buy It, Narcotic Bureau Officials Say Law Gives No Authority to Stop Traffic." The article stated that consumption of marijuana—a "poisonous weed which maddens the senses and emaciates the body of the user" and "the same weed from which the Egyptian hashish is made"—was proceeding "virtually unchecked in Colorado and other Western states with a large Spanish-American population." The article went on to warn that "most crimes of violence in this section, especially in country districts, are laid to users of the drug."[30] That same year a popular Broadway show, *Flying Colors*, included a musical number called "Smokin' Reefers" that called cannabis "the kind of stuff all the dreams are made of" and, perhaps most presciently, "the stuff that white folks are afraid of."

In 1937, Anslinger engineered a blitzkrieg. He had discovered the legend of Hassan-ibn-Sabbah, the Old Man of the Mountain, and he ran with it. Anslinger pointed to Hassan's band of hashish-addled assassins as evidence of marijuana's sinister potential in a widely circulated article in *The American Magazine*, "Marihuana: Assassin of Youth." The article, later made into a movie, claimed that marijuana was a contributing cause in at least two dozen cases of "murder or degenerate sex attacks" and an "alarming wave of sex crime." Anslinger wrote: "How many murders, suicides, robberies, criminal assaults, holdups, burglaries, and deeds of maniacal insanity it causes each year, especially among the young, can be only conjectured. There must be constant enforcement and equally constant education against this enemy, which has a record of murder and terror running through the centuries."[31]

Even though "the more often the story of the Assassins was told, the more ludicrous it became," cannabis historian Ernest L. Abel wrote, it had a powerful effect on the American consciousness. "The image of the demented, knife-wielding, half-crazed hashish user running senseless through the streets, slashing at anyone unfortunate to cross his path, became part of the American nightmare of lawlessness," Abel wrote.[32] The movie *Reefer Madness*, released in 1937, brought the nightmare to the big screen in a soapy film showing adolescents committing murder and rape and going criminally insane after smoking marijuana.

Anslinger pulled out the assassins legend again when he testified before Congress about what he estimated as 50,000 to 100,000 cannabis smokers in the United States, most of them "Negroes and Mexicans and entertainers."[33] Despite counter testimony from the general counsel of the National Institute of Oilseed Products, who said that "millions of people every day are using hempseed in the Orient as food,"[34] and findings by a committee commissioned by New York mayor Fiorello La Guardia that cannabis was neither addictive nor drove users criminally insane, Anslinger's spin became the dominant narrative.

With public sentiment and Congress on his side, Anslinger held a series of secret meetings with Treasury Department officials to draft a law requiring cannabis importers, manufacturers, and sellers to register with the Secretary of the Treasury and pay a prohibitive tax. While the Marihuana Tax Act didn't officially criminalize cannabis, which Anslinger and his crew believed would have been difficult under the terms of the US Constitution, the taxes and red tape it imposed made it nearly impossible for doctors to prescribe it.

"While theoretically the bill was only a means of raising revenue, the real motivation for its enactment is thinly veiled," Lester Grinspoon wrote in *Marihuana Reconsidered.* "By making the individual who wished to smoke *marihuana* pay $100 tax per ounce, the government would effectively force the user to purchase it in an underground market, thereby exposing himself to the risk of tax evasion—an oblique, even in a sense underhanded, attempt at control of the social use of the drug."[35]

The details of the Marihuana Tax Act were held as a closely guarded secret until the day it was presented to the House Ways and Means Committee in 1937. "There was no notification or mention of the predictable effect this legislation would have on the hemp industry or medical profession before the Congressional hearings took place, and the committee members were not alerted to the connection between *marijuana* and hemp; that knowledge would have killed the Marihuana Tax Act dead in its tracks," Robert Deitch wrote in *Hemp: American History Revisited.*[36]

Swayed by Anslinger's testimony and determined to look tough on crime to voters who were growing ever more alarmed about it, Congress passed the act after receiving barely any information and after barely any discussion. In January 1938, the *New York Times* quoted a Treasury Secretary report that said, "The outstanding event of the year in the campaign against drug addiction was the passage of the Federal law placing the traffic in non-tax paid *marijuana* in the same category as other non-tax paid narcotics."[37] Industrial hemp, though non-narcotic, was outlawed by default. Thirteen years later, in 1951, Congress took another big step in cannabis prohibition when it passed the Boggs Act, or Narcotic Drugs Import and Export Act, which penalized cannabis possession like heroin.

Though relatively few people had used cannabis before Anslinger's propaganda blitz, even fewer used it once the Marihuana Tax Act went into effect. Cannabis use remained completely under the radar until it became associated with the counterculture movement of the late 1960s. President Richard M. Nixon unleashed his own antidrug crusade after a 1969 unanimous US Supreme Court decision that the Marihuana Tax Act was unconstitutional because it required suspects to incriminate themselves by paying the tax and assumed (rather than requiring proof) that people who possessed foreign-grown cannabis knew it was smuggled. Nixon responded by calling for harsher penalties for marijuana convictions.

In 1970, Nixon signed the Comprehensive Drug Abuse and Prevention and Control Act, which established "schedules," or categories, for drugs according to their potential for abuse. Cannabis was classified as Schedule 1, along with heroin and LSD, for having no medical potential and the highest potential for abuse. Federal laws imposed a mandatory two- to ten-year sentence for first-time possession of even the smallest amounts of Schedule 1 drugs.[38]

When the National Commission on Marijuana and Drug Abuse, which Nixon appointed in 1972, concluded that marijuana was actually not harmful and should be decriminalized, the president rejected the findings. Nixon's former domestic policy chief John Ehrlichman explained the administration's motivation many years later in a *Harper's* magazine interview. "We knew we couldn't make it illegal to be either against the war or black, but by getting the public to associate the hippies with *marijuana* and blacks with heroin, and then criminalizing both heavily, we could disrupt those communities. We could arrest their leaders, raid their homes, break up their meetings, and vilify them night after night on the evening news. Did we know we were lying about the drugs? Of course we did."[39]

In 1975, the United States began working with Mexico to eradicate cannabis fields with the highly toxic herbicide paraquat, igniting consumer concerns about the safety of cannabis being imported into the United States. Then, President Ronald Reagan and his wife, Nancy, launched the "Just Say No" movement in the 1980s, convincing millions of Americans that cannabis was a menace to society. The Reagan administration imposed harsh mandatory penalties on possession and distribution, and the DEA launched a serious effort to eradicate the outdoor grows that had been planted in the United States, mainly in California and Hawaii. Their continuous slash-and-burn raids are what forced black market cannabis farmers indoors, launching a revolution in "indo" hydroponic growing.

GUNJAH WALLAH: HASH CANDY FOR THE MASSES

In the 1860s, just as books like *The Hasheesh Eater* and *Arabian Nights* were becoming popular in the United States, the Gunjah Wallah Company of New York introduced a hashish-based maple sugar candy that it marketed nationwide through catalogs (including the famous Sears & Roebuck Catalog) and newspaper and magazine ads, including the *Chicago Tribune*, *New York Times*, and *Vanity Fair*. An immediate hit,

Gunjah Wallah candies remained one of the most popular confections in the United States for the next forty years.

A few years after *The Hasheesh Eater* was published, Gunjah Wallah began running advertisements like this one: *The Arabian "Gunjh" of Enchantment confectionized.—A most pleasurable and harmless stimulant.—Cures Nervousness, Weakness, Melancholy, &c. Inspires all classes with new life and energy. A complete mental and physical invigorator.* Price, 25c. and $1 per box, Beware of imitations. Imported only by the *Gunjah-Wallah* Company."

Other ads called the candy "The Great Oriental Nervine Compound," "the theme of song and story among the Persians, Arabians and Assyrians," "a remedy that ought to be in every house on account of its harmlessness and potency," the "true secret of youth and beauty," and a "sure cure" for "general debility and wasting away, all nervous and billios afflictions, torpidity of the liver, croup, hives, colds, coughs, asthma, and incipient consumption."

In an early celebrity endorsement, Confederate General Robert E. Lee endorsed the candy in a full-page ad published in a Boston medical journal, *The Good Samaritan and Domestic Physician*, in the late 1860s or early 1870s. "I wish it was in my power to place a Dollar Box of the HASHEESH CANDY in the pocket of every Confederate Soldier, because I am convinced that it speedily relieves Debility, Fatigue and Suffering," Lee is quoted as saying. The ad gave equal time to the Union, with a quote from General Ulysses S. Grant saying the candy was "of great value for the Wounded and Feeble" and "Harmless." In the same ad, "the celebrated Dr. Mott, of New York" stated that "no doubt but the writings of Mahomet, and the Arabian Night entertainments were produced by writers while under its influence." He went on to say, "I could wish that a Remedy so Potent for good as it is, were more generally in use."

Backlash against the candy was swift and began to appear in the press not long after Gunjah Wallah hit the market. A handful of doctors made it clear they believed the hashish candy was snake oil and the company's miracle-cure claims were false. In 1866, the Philadelphia-based *Medical and Surgical Reporter* ran an editorial about the candy titled "Advertising Quack Medicines."[40] Three years later, the *New York World* ran an article stating that the candies had been "completely discredited."[41]

By the turn of the century, as antihashish propaganda began to shape public sentiment against the confections, the Gunjah Wallah company stopped production.

• 4 •

Pot Brownies and Space Cakes

Poor Alice B. Toklas. Her name will be forever infamous for an autobiography she didn't write (*Autobiography of Alice B. Toklas* was penned by her longtime companion Gertrude Stein) and a brownie recipe she didn't create.

American expatriates Toklas and Stein were at the center of the renaissance in art, music, literature, and cinema that bloomed in Paris in the 1920s, hosting salons that drew intelligentsia from throughout Europe, North Africa, and the Americas. Toklas, a humble and loyal wife, ran the couple's household, edited and typed Stein's manuscripts, prepared their meals on the cook's day off, and sat with the wives while Stein entertained luminaries such as Pablo Picasso and Ernest Hemingway.

An epicurean and an excellent cook, Toklas considered the culinary arts as important as painting or writing and dreamed of one day authoring a cookbook. She finally got to it some twenty years after Stein died, when Toklas was seventy-four years old, under less than ideal circumstances. Battling hepatitis and in need of money, Toklas took on the task of compiling a lifelong collection of recipes and memories alongside her thoughts on French cuisine—in four months.[1]

Running out of time and desperate to make her deadline with Harper & Brothers (the same house that published *The Hasheesh Eater*), Toklas reached out to friends far and wide and asked them to contribute recipes. After Toklas told him that Hemingway was planning to send in a recipe for how to cook a lion (he never did), Brion Gysin, a Canadian artist, poet, and novelist who was living in Tangier, Morocco—and who didn't want to be outdone—sent in a recipe for "Hashish Fudge" as a joke, a way to bridge the gap between Toklas's circle of older bohemians in Paris and Gysin's younger, hipper friends in North Africa.

In his introduction to the recipe, Gysin quipped that the fudge would provide "entertaining refreshment" for a ladies' bridge club or Daughters of the American Revolution meeting and was likely to bring on hysterical fits of laughter and wild floods of thoughts. He also mentioned that obtaining the cannabis for the recipe could be a (not insurmountable) problem because it could often be found growing wild and in city window boxes. Gysin's reference to Baudelaire and the nineteenth-century hash eaters probably should have tipped off Toklas to the prank. Indeed, the recipe is actually not fudge at all, but a basic variation of the majoun that had been enjoyed in India and the Middle East for centuries. (Toklas probably should have been grateful that Gysin left out the Spanish fly and the opium.)

Toklas either never bothered to read Gysin's recipe in her haste or didn't know what cannabis, which Gysin spelled *canibus*, was. Later, she would admit, "It is my ignorance not to have suspected what the few leaves were—of course I didn't know their Latin name."[2] Trusting Gysin as an established writer, Toklas tossed the recipe into her cookbook without editing it. The "fudge" made it into the British edition when the book was published in 1954, but Harper editors in New York caught it and kept it out of the first US edition. Hashish Fudge appears in the second edition released in the early 1960s, probably based on the recipe's popularity overseas. "The recipe was innocently included without my realizing that the hashish was the accented part of the recipe. I was shocked to find that America wouldn't accept it because it was too dangerous," Toklas said in a 1963 interview. "The English are braver. We're not courageous about that sort of thing."[3]

Gysin later told his friends that Toklas took a nibble of the "fudge" once and asked, "Do you think it will take me for a ride?" He was pleased with himself for getting the recipe included. "Alice didn't turn a hair. She rarely did," he said. "I sent it to her feeling it would sell the book, and she badly needed the money."[4]

Toklas's friend, playwright and novelist Thornton Wilder, agreed, telling Toklas that the Hashish Fudge recipe was "the best publicity stunt of the year."[5] It was a bit much for most people in conformist postwar America when the recipe was first published, but by the early 1960s, hipsters were getting hip to Toklas and her culinary tales. In a snide reference to Stein's abstract poetry, *Life* magazine quipped in 1961: "Chief among old culinary belles-lettres in current favor with readers is *The Alice B. Toklas Cook Book*, containing such epicurean nightmares as hashish fudge, undoubtedly for her companion Gertrude Stein's famous hallucination—Pigeon under glass."[6] *Time* was also snide, writing that "the late Poetess Gertrude Stein and her constant companion and autobiographee Alice B. Toklas used to have gay old times together in the kitchen," and suggesting that the inclusion of cannabis could "provide a clue to some of Gertrude Stein's less earthly lines."[7]

The Alice B. Toklas Cook Book, a rich memoir of Parisian bohemian life in the mid-nineteenth century as told from the kitchen, was one of the best-selling cookbooks of all time and deserves a place of honor in the evolution of literary cookery. It will always be remembered, however, for that particular recipe, and the infamous fudge was mentioned in nearly every obituary written about Toklas when she died in 1967. The *New York Times* noted that Toklas had offered a flippant and somewhat cryptic response when asked about it years after the cookbook was published. "What's sauce for the goose may be sauce for the gander," Toklas said. "But it's not necessarily sauce for the chicken, the duck, the turkey, or the guinea hen."[8]

JEREMIAH TOWER, CONSOMMÉ MARIJUANA, AND ALICE AGAIN

Jeremiah Tower, one of the pioneers credited with inventing New American and California cuisine—America's original celebrity chef—can also be credited with throwing the first documented dinner party of the twentieth century featuring cannabis-infused food.

In 1969, when Tower was a student in Cambridge, Massachusetts, he became known around campus for hosting elaborate dinner parties for friends, professors, and guest scholars. He wrote about one of these banquets, held in honor of a visiting poet, in his 2003 memoir, *California Dish: What I Saw (and Cooked) at the American Culinary Revolution.* The menu included Pirozhki, Prosciutto, and Figs, followed by roast beef and then Consommé Marijuana, made from rich chicken stock, fresh basil, sea salt, pepper, and one packed cup of marijuana stems and seeds, strained and served over a chiffonade of nasturtium flowers and basil leaves.

A consummate host who understood timing, Tower served the cannabis broth after the meat and before the watercress salad so it would take effect in time for dessert, and diners could taste strawberries and cream "as we'd never tasted them before," Tower wrote.[9] (Though it's fun to imagine this soup-induced revelry with strawberries, it's not likely it actually could have happened, given the negligible amount of THC in seeds and stems—but there's a lot to be said for the power of suggestion.)

Like many great chefs before him, Tower was also an admirer of Alice B. Toklas and was said to carry a copy of *The Alice B. Toklas Cook Book* with him at all times. In 1975, when he was the chef at Berkeley's famed Chez Panisse, Tower used Toklas's cookbook as the basis for a dinner in honor of what would have been her one hundredth birthday. Hashish Fudge wasn't on the menu.

THE BEATS IN NORTH AFRICA: "LONG MAJOUN PARANTHESES"

In the highly conformist early 1960s, alcohol was America's intoxicant of choice. Anyone who did dare to partake in a different kind of "sauce" generally preferred rolling cannabis into cigarettes rather than eating hash. In a 1962 article, "The Prodigal Powers of Pot," *Playboy* writer Dan Wakefield wrote: "In other parts of the world cannabis is often eaten (Hindu ladies munch it in a candy called *majoon*, and Mexicans sometimes mix it in their chili) as well as drunk (Haitians are among those who brew it as a tea). But Americans prefer to smoke it in cigarettes, and have generally shunned suggested variations, such as Gertrude Stein's recipe for Marijuana Fudge." (He was confused about the recipe's authorship, of course, but Toklas was likely used to that.)

These smokers, the first in a demographic cluster of progressive professionals that would later be called "cultural creatives," were from the middle class, Wakefield wrote. They were "not the Rotarian wing of the middle class, but the branch that brings back Olympia Press books from Europe, prefers Medaglia d'Oro to Maxwell House, and works in what is known as the communications field."[10] (Think Peggy Olson smoking a joint as she types furiously in the TV series *Mad Men*.)

For the most part, however, hashish, cannabis, and other mind-altering substances remained the realm of fringe artists, writers, and poets known as Beats (derogatorily, Beatniks), successors to Toklas's bohemian salon set and predecessors to the hippies. Gysin, a major figure in the Beat movement (though like many of his compatriots, he refused to be called one), also became fascinated with Hassan-ibn-Sabbah, the Old Man of the Mountain, while he was an expat in Morocco, and even named his restaurant in Tangier 1001 Nights. He shared his love for majoun, the food of the assassins, with fellow expats, putting dynamite to their rebellious creativity.

Writer Paul Bowles told *Rolling Stone* he went on a majoun binge to resolve the death scene in *The Sheltering Sky*, his bleak 1949 novel about a New York couple drifting from city to city in the North African desert, a book that Norman Mailer later said "opened up the world of Hip" to "let in the murder, the drugs, the incest, the death of the Square . . . the call of the orgy, the end of civilization."[11] Writer and artist William S. Burroughs also enjoyed majoun during his time in Tangier, where he penned his famous novel *Naked Lunch* and once wrote a letter home explaining that he was working on "long majoun parentheses."[12]

Burroughs picked up on and shared Gysin's fascination with the legend of the eleventh-century assassins, which showed up periodically in his work. (Burroughs claimed that Gysin was the reincarnation of Hassan, but Gysin rejected the idea because he wanted to be known as "the man from nowhere.") In his poem condemning the evils of covert intelligence agencies and big business, "The Last Words of Hasan I Sabbah," Burroughs wrote: "You want Hassan Sabbah to tidy that up? You've got the wrong number." Hasan's legendary last words—"nothing is true, everything is permitted," which became known as the Assassin's Creed—were the perfect motto for the rebellious Beats (and the title of Gysin's biography, published in 2005).

Portrayed in the media as disrespectful, slovenly, and lazy, "Beatniks"—and the drugs associated with them—were generally disliked and ridiculed in mainstream America, represented in the media by goofy characters like Maynard G. Krebs, the goateed, unkempt sidekick in the early 1960s sitcom *The Many Loves of Dobie Gillis*.

The media portrayed a more frightening side to the movement for conformity-craving Americans as well. In a 1959 *Life* magazine feature on the Beats, writer Paul O'Neil said they had "raised their voices against virtually every aspect of current American society: Mom, Dad, Politics, Marriage, the Savings Bank, Organized Religion, Literary Elegance, Law, the Ivy League Suit and Higher Education, to say nothing of the Automatic Dishwasher, the Cellophane-wrapped Soda Cracker, the Split-Level House and the clean, or peace-provoking, H-bomb."

O'Neil described the "Beatnik" as "a hot-eyes fellow in beard and sandals, or a 'chick' with scraggly hair, long black stockings, heavy eye make-up and an expression which could indicate either hauteur or uneasy digestion," someone who admired "the Negro" for his "irresponsibility, cheerful promiscuity and subterranean defiance which were once enforced in him during his years of bondage." None of this was acceptable in the repressed and racist 1950s, but perhaps even more terrifying, O'Neil wrote that Beats partook of terrifying drugs that propelled them to depravity and the brink of insanity. He held up Burroughs, who "dosed himself with alcohol, heroin, marijuana, *kif*, majoun, and a hashish candy," as a prime example.[13]

In 1961, poet, photographer, underground filmmaker, and publisher Ira Cohen hopped the same Hungarian freighter that Jack Kerouac had jumped a year earlier to meet up with Gysin, Burroughs, Bowles, and the rest of the gang in Tangier. He, too, discovered majoun and fell victim to its charms. Cohen became something of an ambassador for hashish and majoun among the expats in Morocco, and he could often be found holding court in restaurants and bars around Tangier, wearing long, dark robes and offering Westerners elaborate instructions in how to prepare the confection.

About five years later, Cohen decided it was time to share the delights of majoun with the masses. Through his book imprint, Gnaoua Press, he published *The Hashish Cookbook*, a slim volume of cannabis-infused recipes written by "Panama Rose," in 1966. Cohen was widely and erroneously credited with writing the book, which was actually penned by his then-girlfriend, Rosalind, who was known professionally by her first name only. The twenty-page book included recipes for traditional favorites such as bhang and majoun as well as some don't-try-this-at-home recipes playfully reminiscent of the Assassins and *Club des Hashischin*: an aphrodisiac made from mace, red saffron, Grains of Paradise, and cantharides beetles (Spanish fly) and a skin salve calling for human (or chicken) fat, hashish, Indian hemp, belladonna, and opium poppy flowers.

Panama Rose borrowed from the nomadic tribes of Morocco's Rif Mountains for Nebuchadnezzar's Dream, a recipe that involved toasting whole cannabis stalks over an open fire and dipping them in salt and honey, and offered a cannabis-infused version of the Moroccan soup that was traditionally served to break the Ramadan fast. The *Hashish Cookbook* suggested adding toasted cannabis seeds to fritters "for a weird breakfast" and included perhaps the first real documented recipe for pot brownies with the recipe for Hash Brownies, which noted that "hashish and chocolate are a fine combination."

The author warned that the brownies should be cut into tiny squares and nibbled with caution and suggested counteracting "any unpleasant side effect resulting from overindulgence, such as severe paranoia," with cold fresh lemonade, bed rest, and warm blankets (advice that has been repeated, in one form or another, down through the ages).

Cohen printed ten thousand copies of *The Hashish Cookbook* in 1966, and they sold out in six weeks. That same year, he wrote "The Goblet of Dreams," an ode to majoun in *Playboy* magazine that introduced many young Americans to the delights of the Moroccan confection as well as Hassan-ibn-Sabbah, "the legendary old man of the mountain who led his cult of assassins from Mount Alamut in Persia and certainly one of the most renowned of all hashish eaters." Cohen wrote that in Morocco, "the special confection with Indian hemp, or kif, as its main ingredient" was "as commonplace as fruitcake in England or angel-food cake in the United States," available "any time you feel like traveling or crave some instant magic theater." Cohen described majoun as gummy, greenish-black sticks about the size of a thumb that were made from the cannabis plant's resin or powdered buds and flowers and said they were readily available in Moroccan marketplaces. They were usually taken, he said, "on festive nights or in the wintertime, when it keeps you warm through the long Moroccan nights."

Sounding much like his hash-eating predecessors of a century earlier, Cohen described the experience of eating majoun—which he said could last for up to twenty-four hours—in various terrifying yet exhilarating ways: descending into unknown depths surrounded by hundreds of shining eyes; being embedded in black tar while he glowed like sapphires; leaving his body behind and soaring through the air holding on for dear life. For the most part, Cohen wrote that the experiences would culminate in oceans of laughter. "It is the same as it has been for many centuries, and the Thousand and One Nights happened just yesterday, are still happening around you, whole there in the center of colors, the storyteller unfolds his tale of the miraculous Aladdin who was conceived in majoon," Cohen wrote.

Enjoying a piece of majoun made Moorish women dreamy and sensual, he continued, "though they say it makes them want to take off all their clothes and run naked through the streets." That was likely not because of the hashish in the confection, however, as Cohen attributed majoun's reputation as "an erotic electuary" to the use of Spanish fly in the recipe. Because of that ingredient, Cohen promised *Playboy* readers that properly made majoun would "set the stage for a night of *houris* (virgins) and exotic delights, for Allah is all-merciful and will provide endless orgasm in paradise." And again, that warning to nibble slowly, with a caveat: "You have nothing to lose but yourself, and that is precisely what you may find in the losing."[14]

In a letter to the editor three months later, renowned American psychologist Timothy Leary, who had been dismissed from the Harvard University Department of Psychology three years earlier for failing to observe established research guidelines in his studies of psychedelic drugs, wrote a letter to *Playboy* applauding Cohen's article for providing valuable historical and sociological perspective. "*Playboy* and Ira Cohen do us a favor by reminding us that Eastern and Middle Eastern cultures—older, holier, wiser and sensually more mature than our own—have used psychedelic plants for thousands of years; not for rebellious kicks (a depressingly vulgar American concept), but for thoughtful, aesthetically precise, delicately managed ecstatic experiences," Leary wrote.[15]

I LOVE YOU, ALICE B. TOKLAS! GROOVY BROWNIES FROM A FREAKY COOKBOOK

Ira Cohen and the rest of his crew of writers and artists who congregated in Morocco in the 1950s and 1960s opened up a whole new world for young Americans with their descriptions of life along the Hashish Trail—the region that Marco Polo made famous, spanning from Turkey and Lebanon to Morocco, Spain, and France—home to the world's major hash-producing centers.

For the next ten years or so, just before the region erupted in widespread political violence and wars that would prevent most Westerners from vacationing in Baghdad or Kandahar for the next decades, hippies carrying worn paperback copies of *One Thousand and One Nights* in their tie-dyed shoulder bags swarmed to places they knew based only on the names of the hash they smoked at home (Afghani, Kashmir, Pakistani), seeking freely available hashish and majoun. Hotels, restaurants, and bus services cropped up along the route to service the Westerners along the Hashish Trail, who kept each other informed via clandestine networks and the underground press. The travelers brought the recipes for the hashish food they encountered home with them, adopting the Indian and Middle Eastern recipes to please the palates of their fellow Americans and introducing many to the delights of taking cannabis "out of the joint or pipe and into the kitchen," Lester Grinspoon wrote.[16]

This was, to say the least, alarming to mainstream America. On the eve of the Summer of Love, most Americans who had read about Leary and his friends' experiments with drugs were leery. Mainstream Americans still saw marijuana-loving Beats, who had morphed almost overnight into hippies, as slightly dangerous caricatures to be marginalized and monitored. A 1966 *Life* magazine article, "Mad New Scene on Sunset Strip," described a disturbingly free-spirited society "based on love with plenty of marijuana for all."[17]

Less than a year later, in an article declaring the underground art movement a wild utopian dream, *Life* warned that stores were popping up in major cities everywhere to sell incense, water pipes, mandala charts, and "things to improve your trip," while several underground newspapers were publishing "homemakers' columns that give recipes for hashish cookies, aspic of mescaline, 'pot-seed pancakes for a groovy breakfast high.'"[18]

A few months later, *Life* declared an epidemic. In "Marijuana: Millions of Turned-On Users," it reported that marijuana, "a mild euphoric drug known and used throughout much of the world for centuries and long a part of the bohemian scene in the U.S., suddenly has become commonplace on college campuses, among intellectuals and suburbanites, and—most worrisome of all—even among subteenagers." Encouraged by rock 'n' roll groups, underground newspapers, and "psychedelic shops," *Life* warned, vulnerable teens were being led "into a drug-culture shadow world and on to a psychological dependence whose implications for users—and for society—are disturbing indeed."

Even though the crime rate in hippie communities was astonishingly low, aside from their massive violation of drug laws, and hippies were "embarrassingly full of love" when arrested, *Life* spied an insurrection. "It remains to be seen how socially damaged they will become by living in such outright violation of both law and cultural taboo," the magazine noted.[19]

In 1968, the year between the Summer of Love and Woodstock, the Motion Picture Producers and Distributors of America reflected the new era of free love, drugs, and rock and roll that was emerging in the country when it officially lifted the Hays Code, a 1930 self-regulation edict censoring everything from sex to profanity to drug and alcohol use in movies, which was enacted after Hollywood drew the ire of religious and temperance groups such as Legion of Decency. Enforcement of the Hays Code had been unraveling throughout the 1960s, but with its girdle fully unsnapped, celluloid psychedelia exploded.

Cannabis, along with LSD and cocaine, landed firmly in the American cinemascape as both muse and new-age plot hook. It was the dawn of the "stoner movie," with The Monkees' *Head*, which set the stage for a genre of weird rock band movies; The Beatles' fantastical animated motion picture *Yellow Submarine*, which Beat writer Ken Kesey said "looks better stoned, but that's true of all movies";[20] and Stanley Kubrick's *2001: A Space Odyssey*, the sci-fi classic that spawned conspiracy theories about Kubrick faking the moon landing and the first movie to be marketed directly to a new and quickly expanding class of cannabis users.

Also released that year was the film that put the pot brownie on the map for most Americans and the first major motion picture to make cannabis an integral part of the plot—truly, the first stoner movie, and yet another nut in the majoun of Alice B. Toklas's mistaken identity. *I Love You, Alice B. Toklas!* starred Peter Sellers as Harold Fine, a dissatisfied suburban Los Angeles lawyer who bumbles through an unlikely plot with a sitar-laden soundtrack that involves eating cannabis-laced brownies and leaving his aging secretary-fiancée at the altar to drop out with Nancy, a beautiful hippie with a butterfly tattoo, while somehow managing to represent the reactions taking place in many Americans' hearts and minds to the deep cultural changes that were blowing up in 1968. It was in this movie that the poorly named Hashish Fudge from Toklas's cookbook was forever transformed into the pot brownie, and the pot brownie became synonymous with Toklas's name.

In the film's pivotal scene, Nancy dumped her cannabis stash into the bowl of an electric mixer along with fudge brownie mix and eggs, mixed up a batch, left Harold a note about the "groovy brownies," and split. Harold, not understanding what "groovy" meant, shared the brownies with his parents and fiancée, who found them delicious, resulting in an exaggerated intoxication scene reminiscent of the 1937 propaganda film *Reefer Madness*, in which the parents laughed hysterically and Harold's fiancé ripped off his clothes and begged him to take her. Later, when Harold berated Nancy for not telling him what was in the brownies, she said, "Thank Alice B. Toklas. It was her recipe. She wrote a freaky cookbook."

For better or worse, the brownie trip changed Harold's life. He left Joyce at the altar, grew his hair long (seemingly overnight), lived for a while with Nancy in his car, then moved back home, got annoyed about her friends and free love, got back together with ex-fiancée Joyce, and left her at the altar again. The movie ended with Harold running out of the synagogue, yelling that there's got to be something beautiful out there. Try as she might, Harold's mother was never able to find the bakery that made the delicious brownies so she can pick up some more.

With its light, breezy soundtrack (in the same year as *Yellow Submarine*) and its campy hippie jokes, *I Love You, Alice B. Toklas!* got mixed reviews. Critic Roger Ebert found the movie's representation of hippies—people who "wear funny clothes, sleep on the stove, don't

Julia Asked Alice

A few summers after Julia Child arrived in Paris in 1948, she invited Alice B. Toklas to dinner at her apartment. Child spent two days preparing *ballottine* of veal with Madeira truffle sauce. Toklas, a tiny woman whose face could barely be seen under the large hat she wore, never tasted it. She stayed for a glass of wine and left.

Feeding Frenzies on Film

I Love You, Alice B. Toklas! was the first major motion picture that used cannabis, and in particular cannabis-laced food, as an important part of the plot line, and it remained the only one of any note until the twenty-first century, when cannabis laws began to be relaxed and more people were introduced to cannabis food. Smoking cannabis was still much more prevalent in films, but in the 2000s edibles began to show up on screen.

Saving Grace (2000): Two matronly ladies brew a pot of tea using leaves they didn't know were cannabis, and hilarity involving cornflakes and funny glasses ensues. Later, the heroine lights her cannabis harvest on fire and gets an entire village high, à la the Scythians.

Smiley Face (2007): A struggling actress accidentally eats a batch of cannabis cupcakes and spends a madcap day of misadventures trying to get to a hemp festival in Venice Beach to pay off her dealer, whom she is convinced is going to take her only valuable possession, a Sleep Number bed.

Adventureland (2009): An amusement park worker cheers up his coworkers with pot brownies, then gets into an altercation with some angry dudes.

High School (2010): The adventures of a high school valedictorian who, fearing he might fail a drug test and lose his scholarship, serves the entire school cannabis-laced brownies so everyone else would fail the test, too.

Hall Pass (2011): A group of middle-aged friends overindulges in pot brownies on the golf course and ends up doing snow angels and defecating in the sand traps.

Newlyweeds (2013): Critically received indie flick in which a Brooklyn woman's downfall comes when children who live next door steal hashish brownies from her bag and freak out.

The Boss (2016): A woman who just got out of jail employs Girl Scouts to sell cannabis-laced chocolate edibles outside a Chicago medical marijuana dispensary.

wash, read the Los Angeles *Free Press*, bake pot brownies, put up posters everywhere, and operate with a sort of mindless, directionless love ethic"—conventional,[21] but *Variety* called it "a sympathetic look at the advantages and disadvantages" of both hippie life and "what is considered 'normal' modes of behavior."[22]

"A comedy of pre-conditioned effects" is what *New York Times* critic Vincent Canby called *I Love You, Alice B. Toklas!*. "By the end of it," Canby wrote, "I was feeling a certain amount of resentment at having been had, along with Alice B. Toklas, whose name, apparently, is to become an automatic laugh, like smog and girdle."[23]

Toklas died the year before the movie bearing her name was released, but Gysin was delighted when he found out that the plot revolved around the recipe he had sent his old friend so many years ago. Ever in need of money, Gysin contacted the film's producers to see if there were any way to milk some money or publicity out of it. Though he tried, Brion Gysin Hashish Fudge never stuck.[24] The pot brownie would be attached to Toklas, who may or may not have ever eaten one, forevermore.

THE NETHERLANDS: SPACE CAKES AND A BACKDOOR PROBLEM

By luck of geography, with its unparalleled access to shipping lanes on the North Sea that open up to the world's markets and resources, The Netherlands has always been an important gateway for commerce and transport, attracting traders from around the world. The densely populated country, where vast amounts of wealth were accumulated from opium and tobacco, was naturally tolerant of the hashish introduced by trading partners in North Africa, but not many Dutch people used it until small groups of painters, writers, and musicians picked it up in the 1950s. More people began using it throughout the turbulent 1960s, when smoking hash at the national monument in Dam Square or the Vondelpark in Amsterdam became a pilgrimage of sorts for both local and visiting hippies. By the end of the decade, the number of cannabis users in The Netherlands was estimated to be between ten thousand and fifteen thousand.[25]

Among those were the crème de la crème of the American Beat generation, including poets Allen Ginsberg and Gregory Corso, who discovered Amsterdam's flourishing hashish scene in the early 1960s and became fixtures in the city's jazz cafés. In Amsterdam, though hashish and cannabis were technically illegal, laws were rarely enforced until the mid-1960s, after the United States and Germany pressured The Netherlands into joining the UN Single Convention on Narcotic Drugs of 1961. At the same time, the counterculture movement was taking hold in The Netherlands, and the cloud of cannabis smoke hanging over Vondelpark became one of their more powerful symbols. As a form of nonviolent protest, Robert Jasper Grootveld, the leader of a revolutionary group called Provo, grew cannabis on the roof of his Amsterdam houseboat—and got away with it.[26]

For the Dutch, cannabis seemed a nonissue compared to the massive problems that drugs like heroin and cocaine began to cause in the late 1960s, an epidemic that was seeping beyond the country's borders and angering its neighbors. The Dutch did not prescribe to the widely held theory, promoted by the United States, that cannabis was a gateway drug leading users to take up harder ones. Lacking the resources to enforce laws against all drugs equally and recognizing that "soft" drugs like cannabis were not nearly as dangerous as "hard" drugs like heroin, in 1969 the government adopted a characteristically practical drug policy of "cooperation despite differences" known as *Gedogen*, which tolerates and even permits illegal activity. In a show of solidarity with the policy, in 1970 the police very publicly stood amid the crowd in plain clothes as people lit up around them during the Kralingen Holland Pop Festival, a 1970 Woodstock-like concert in Rotterdam.

Gedogen was formalized in the revised Opium Act in 1976, which cracked down hard on substances with "unacceptable risk to the health of the user" and promoted tolerance for cannabis products. The Opium Act revisions led to decriminalization and allowed the government to regulate, tax, and monitor legitimate retail sales and use of cannabis, with a goal of keeping cannabis users away from the hard drugs sold on the streets and giving rise to an industry based around "coffee shops" that sold cannabis, hashish, and cannabis-laced food alongside coffee and pastries. A. C. M. Jansen, an economist who spent more than four hundred hours studying Dutch coffee houses in 1991, found that the Dutch strategy was successful in keeping people away from harder drugs,[27] but in an effort to stay within the confines of the 1961 Single Convention on Narcotic Drugs, The Netherlands didn't legalize—and actually increased penalties for—production and large-scale distribution of cannabis, leaving fully legal and licensed coffee shops reliant on the black market for their product and creating what is known as "the backdoor problem."

In the swinging 1960s and 1970s, Amsterdam was one of the epicenters of a burgeoning global cannabis culture, swarming with hippies and freaks who were drawn to the city that *Newsweek* declared "the drug, sex and do-your-thing capital of the Western world." In a 1971 *Playboy* article declaring Amsterdam "youth mecca of the world," Reg Potterton described a place "where city council members said dope should be legalized and had themselves photographed in front of city hall, zonked out and glassy-eyed, waving hash bombers at the cameras," and the Council for Youth Education called for fixed-price cannabis products sold at drug stores. At Paradiso and Fantasia, "two shabby old buildings that the city council subsidizes to the tune of $50,000 a year," patrons could consume cannabis, drink beer or soda, and "watch avant-garde theatrical productions or nude ballets, listen to music, paint, sculpt, sing, shout, dance, make out and turn on," Potterton wrote. The current price and availability of hash was reported weekly on the state-controlled radio, followed by police warnings about the hazards of switching from soft to hard drugs.[28]

A hippie named Wernard Bruining paved the way for the new industry when he and a group of friends opened the first coffee shop—which Bruining called a tea house after the hashish joints popular in the United States in the 1920s and 1930s—in a former bakery they were squatting in on Weesperzijde in 1972. They named the place Mellow Yellow, after a Donovan song about a yellow vibrator, and they sold cannabis flowers and hash smuggled in from Morocco, Afghanistan, and Turkey as well as cannabis-infused confections known as "space cakes." After a fire destroyed the bakery building in 1978, Mellow Yellow moved to a prime location on Vijzelstraat, between the Heineken Brewery and Rembrandt Square, where it was one of Amsterdam's most popular tourist attractions until it closed on December 31, 2016. (In the early 1980s, Bruining grew tired of running cannabis for his shop through Zurich, so he teamed up with a group of Americans to breed and clone new strains that could thrive in The Netherlands, which he called "Netherweed." It never caught on in the sun-stricken country.)

Henk de Vries, a drug smuggler who got his start peddling hash in matchboxes at the 1970 Kralingen festival as the police looked the other way to prove their tolerance, became Bruining's first competitor in 1975 when he opened The Bulldog in his late father's sex store in Amsterdam's red-light district. On its website, The Bulldog claims de Vries invented the term "coffee shop as we know it today for Amsterdam," and the first Bulldog's living room–like atmosphere, where people talked, drank, and played board and card games, embodied the term.[29] As the cannabis industry blossomed in Amsterdam throughout the 1970s and 1980s, The Bulldog grew with it. De Vries moved the operation into a former police headquarters on the Leidseplein and built his popular multilevel coffee shop and retail store into a multimillion-dollar empire (see photo below).

Coffee shops were as common in Amsterdam in the 1980s as Starbucks would be in every city in the next decade. In Amsterdam in particular, they evolved from rundown cafés in shady backstreets into bright, lively meeting places with natural light and ferns in prominent locations. In 1986—the year that *High Times* writer Simon Vinkenoog recorded his amazement that the 1960s spirit had survived in Amsterdam into the 1980s and wondered whether that could be considered "a futuristic signpost for other societies to follow suit"[30]—The Netherlands was home to an estimated six hundred coffee shops where cannabis and hashish were openly sold and consumed, 350 of them

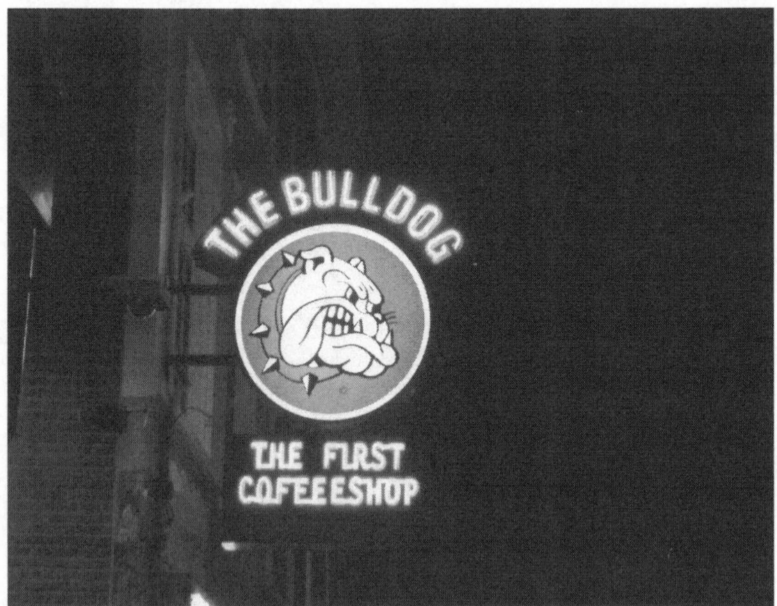

The Bulldog Café in Amsterdam. Photo by Chris Kilham.

in Amsterdam.[31] The city was a magnet for cannabis-seeking tourists who didn't have many other places to go in the 1980s and early 1990s, as a new round of global drug crackdowns and political violence shut down other options.

By 1994, the Dutch people had had enough of the coffee shop scene. The government was overrun with citizens' complaints that the industry attracted too many noisy tourists, particularly in towns along borders with France and Germany. It responded with a set of official regulations for the coffee shops, setting the legal age to buy cannabis at eighteen, restricting loitering and noise, limiting sales to no more than thirty grams of cannabis or cannabis products at coffee shops, and capping each coffee shop's allowable stock at five hundred grams.

The new policies also allowed local municipalities to prohibit or restrict coffee shops, which many did. The number of coffee shops nationwide dropped from about 1,500 in the mid-1990s to 846 in the late 1990s.[32] Many of the seedier establishments targeted at tourists from neighboring countries were weeded out, making way for what *High Times* called "a new breed of cannabis-friendly environments where professors and poets can mingle with politicians and police."[33]

"Drug tourism" in The Netherlands was certainly not dead. In 1996, it was believed to account for 25 percent of the country's tourism income, with taxable annual revenue between $300 billion and $400 billion.[34] Upscale coffee shop owners knew how to appeal to the new batch of upper-demographic tourists who came seeking their wares, and it could be hard to distinguish between coffee shops that just sold coffee and "real" ones like Greenhouse Effect, a coffee shop with Santa Fe–style décor in Amsterdam's red-light district that author and activist Michael Pollan described in a 1995 *New York Times Magazine* article as offering fruit drinks, snacks, "an alarming-looking psychoactive pastry called 'space cake,' and a dozen different kinds of cannabis and hashish, sold by the gram or the joint."

In Amsterdam, Pollan found "a community of émigré Americans that revolves around the culture of marijuana in much the same way earlier communities of emigres in Europe sprang up around avant-garde literature or painting while awaiting acceptance at home."[35] Much like the artists and writers who gathered to stimulate each other's creativity and pick each other's brains at Toklas's and Stein's salons, this expat community—made up largely of refugees from the war on drugs, drawn to The Netherlands' reputation for tolerance—shared ideas and innovations about cannabis and, in particular, indoor growing. They created a revolution in the supply chain as domestic production overtook imports to stock coffee shop shelves in the 1980s. As more and more coffee shops replaced their inventory from North Africa with indo-grown strains known as Eurocannabis, growers in The Netherlands pushed technology and drove hydroponic cultivation into new realms. Production exploded. During the "Green Avalanche" of the 1990s, domestic growers captured 80 percent of the cannabis market in The Netherlands.[36]

In the early twenty-first century, the government took another hardline stance against the cannabis industry, which had proliferated massively again during the 1990s. By 2001, the industry encompassed between 1,200 and 1,500 coffee shops selling cannabis and hashish, 350 to 450 of them in Amsterdam,[37] and was estimated to be worth between $360 million and $1.1 billion, employed between three thousand and four thousand workers, and even had its own union, the *Bond van Cannabis Detaillisten*.[38] Unhappy with this image and getting pressure from France and Belgium, where much of The Netherlands' cannabis supply was ending up, the Dutch government beefed up its prosecution of growers and implemented a system that allowed cannabis to be sold only to Dutch citizens. Amsterdam city officials, fearing a catastrophic loss of tourist income, made a deal with the national government that allowed it to override the so-called Weed Pass in return for cracking down on regulations such as coffee shops' proximity to schools—which it did.

By 2018, the number of coffee shops in Amsterdam had dropped to 167, and after forty-five years in business, Mellow Yellow, the pioneering tea house, was not among them. The world's first coffee shop was shut down for being within 250 meters of a hair-styling school, a development many in the industry saw as an omen of things to come. August de Loor, the founder of *Bond van Cannabis Detaillisten*, told the *Telegraph* that the "most negative scenario" was that coffee shops could disappear entirely within five to ten years.[39]

As other countries steadily reformed their own cannabis laws, they learned from The Netherlands' mistakes and implemented regulatory systems without the backdoor problem. Hungry for the billions of dollars being brought in by the cannabis industry, cities from Barcelona to Tbilisi rushed in to declare themselves "the new Amsterdam."

Chocolate and Cannabis: A Fine Pairing

Cacao beans, revered since ancient times as food and medicine, have long been considered an aphrodisiac, perhaps because they contain tryptophan, a serotonin booster, and phenylethylamine, a stimulant related to amphetamine. The Aztec emperor Montezuma was said to drink one hundred cups of chocolate a day. The Olmecs of southern Mexico fermented, roasted, and ground cacao beans for consuming (usually drinking) as early as 1500 BC. In the sixteenth century, Spanish conquistador Hernán Cortéz wrote to Spain's King Carlos I about *xovoatl*, a cacao drink said to build up resistance and fight fatigue. Cacao made its way to Spain and across Europe, where it became the preferred morning and bedtime drink of the upper classes.

Many chefs and scientists believe chocolate and cannabis are an ideal pairing, not only because chocolate masks the hashy flavor but also because the two share chemical cousins, THC and anandamide, that affect appetite, mood, and pain perception. THC, probably the most famous molecule in cannabis, agonizes cannabinoid receptors in the human body, causing psychoactive and medical effects. Anandamide, a lipid produced in the human brain that is also found in chocolate, is nearly chemically identical to THC and brings on a very mild, some say imperceptible, high. When THC and anandamide double team, scientists believe, they could inhibit the breakdown of cannabinoids THC and CBD, causing them to stay in the system longer and enhancing their benefits.

What this means is, most people get higher and stay high longer when they combine cannabis and chocolate. That's one reason the pot brownie has endured.

HIGH TIMES: MAJOUN AGAIN, CHEF RA'S CULINARY TRIPS, AND SUGAR SPINS

It's a success story every magazine publisher dreams about. In 1974, Thomas King Forçade (born Kenneth Gary Goodson)—a radical activist who made his living smuggling ganja from Jamaica to Florida and had tried, and failed, several times to publish underground newspapers and magazines—printed the first issue of *High Times* magazine as a joke. The black-and-white cover showed a woman lifting a mushroom (presumably psilocybin) suggestively to her lips, and the cover lines promised articles inside about hemp paper, "a lady dealer," and Timothy Leary's "ultimate trip."

Forçade intended the magazine to be a one-off parody of *Playboy*, with glamour shots and a centerfold photo of voluptuous cannabis plants instead of women (a harbinger, perhaps, of the "Miss *High Times*" feature that would come later). Forçade was as surprised as anyone when more than half a million copies sold, and readers wanted more.[40] Figuring he might as well crank out a few monthly issues, Forçade recruited heavyweight writers he knew from his failed newspapers, including gonzo journalist Hunter S. Thompson and Beat writers William Burroughs and Allen Ginsberg to pen feature articles. The magazines kept getting better. For four years, circulation doubled with every issue until *High Times* hit its peak of four million readers in 1978—the same year Forçade shot himself in his New York City apartment at the age of thirty-three.

That was also the year that *High Times* introduced its readers to majoun, in a feature article titled "Eat It!" by J. F. Burke, who described the hash candy as having "the consistency of nougat, or perhaps a little softer, with a bouquet of scents." Burke had experienced his first psychedelic trip with majoun when he was a sailor in the 1930s, and he offered up his recipe: Mix crumbled hashish with raw sugar and powdered arrowroot, add sweet butter and mix thoroughly, then add a little honey and chopped, unsalted pistachios. While Burke declared pure hash "a delicacy, a gustatory delight," he said it was hard to come by in the United States, and additives such as pitch, camphor, spices, datura, henbane, and opium were common. "I have often thought that the nightmarish experiences reported by Baudelaire, Gautier, and many others could be attributed to Datura and/or henbane in their hashish," he wrote.

For readers who weren't interested in majoun, Burke offered an array of ways to use cannabis in the kitchen. "You can eat a little grass as a digestive, eat more for a stimulant, or eat still more as an intoxicant," Burke wrote, but he warned that "eating raw grass is rather like eating fodder." Burke advised readers to simply add cannabis or hash to any brownie recipe; throw a handful of manicured tops into soup, stew, or salad; or add raw cannabis to soups, stews, salads, pastries, or candies.

And if readers ate too much? "You'll be drunk," Burke stated. "You may barf. You might trip. But you won't die. The lethal dose of THC would be 4,000,000 milligrams, a rather unwieldy mass to get into one's stomach, much less keep there."[41]

After Forçade's death, *High Times* lost its way, struggling for footing and focusing more on cocaine than cannabis. In the mid-1980s, just as indoor growing was beginning to take off in the United States and around the world, John Howell and Steve Hager took over and refocused the magazine. *High Times* boasted that it taught "tokers the world over how to grow their own high-quality pot at home,"[42] and with the debut of Chef Ra's "Psychedelic Kitchen" column, the magazine helped them cook with it on a regular basis as well.

Hager hired his high school friend Jim Wilson, who took the name Chef Ra, to write about cannabis-infused food in a column called "Psychedelic Kitchen," which *High Times* introduced in 1988 with a cover photo of Chef Ra holding a big plate of vegetables. It was one of the magazine's best-selling issues, and for the next fifteen years, Chef Ra delivered on his promise of "a culinary trip, cuisine for the mind and body" with his cannabis-infused recipes. Over the years, he published recipes influenced by both Southern and Jamaican *ital* cookery, everything from Puna Butter (a half ounce of "sensi" and two sticks of butter, heated in a skillet until the butter is dark and tastes like butterscotch) to festive dishes such as Ganjaween Grilled Apples in Dips and a Worldwide *High Times* Thanksgiving Feast.

Chef Ra wrote that he began cooking with cannabis after he was turned on to none other than Alice B. Toklas's brownie recipe, though it was pretty clear he hadn't read her actual cookbook. "This hippie chef had the right idea about how to cook," he wrote. "I started creating marijuana-laced recipes that produced different kinds of highs because of the various strains of pot used. I would get Jamaican and Mexican weeds that produced the 'up-ahead' sativa high when eaten. On the other hand, Panama Red, Colombian Red Bud, and Gold Mexican produced a 'smackdown' high where all you wanted to do was lie on the bed. And when Nevil from Seed Bank showed up from Amsterdam with all those bomb-ass indica strains, you knew better than to go operating any heavy machinery after consuming."[43]

Chef Ra died in his sleep in 2006. Ashley Boudreaux, a New Orleans chef, took over the food column for a couple of years, and the magazine published recipes from contributing chefs such as Mike DeLao, Scott Durrah, and Herb Seidel (and a few guys with names like Easy Bake Dave) until 2015, when longtime staffer Elise McDonough, who had been styling recipes for photo shoots and writing food articles as a passion project, was named edibles editor. In 2012, McDonough's collection of the magazine's best recipes through the years, *The Official High Times Cannabis Cookbook*, had made history as the first professionally produced cannabis cookbook to be published by a major publisher, Chronicle Books.

In July 2016, food was back on the *High Times* cover again with McDonough's article, "Ganja Gourmet" and a photo of cannabis flower and vegetable shish kebabs. McDonough told of sitting next to *Los Angeles Times* restaurant critic Jonathan Gold at a secret cannabis dinner four years earlier and described a dynamic fine dining scene that had evolved since then. With help from Laurie Wolf and Melissa Parks, authors of the newly released *Herb: Mastering the Art of Cooking with Cannabis*, McDonough offered recipes for Cannabis-Infused Bacon-Wrapped Dates, Creamy Butternut Squash Soup, Bucatini with Sour Diesel, Cannachurri Steak Kebabs, and Bannabis Cream Pie.

McDonough's interview in that same issue with chef, TV star, and rapper Action Bronson, host of *Fuck, That's Delicious!* on Viceland, was indicative of the turn cannabis cuisine was taking. Bronson said he was a huge fan of cannabis-infused edibles, but he didn't eat the sugary ones because "eating a fudge bar filled with sugar, that makes you fucking crash. It makes you spin. . . . it makes me spin. When a lot of people take edibles, I think it's the reaction of the sugar with the THC that really fucks 'em, because that shit sends you down a winding path that's not good. It's kind of like being high and drunk—it's too much, you know."[44]

McDonough left *High Times* in 2017 after a group of investors including reggae star Bob Marley's son Damian bought a controlling interest in the magazine for $70 million, promising to "build on the strong base they created to bring *High Times* from the authority in the counterculture movement to a modern media enterprise."[45] She contributed to another cookbook, *Bong Appétit: Mastering the Art of Cooking with Weed*, published by Penguin Random House in 2018, and continued to write about an industry she saw at a tipping point.

"For many years when I was judging the Cannabis Cup, the quality of the edibles was pretty much the same, and all the packaging was pretty plain. In the last couple years, that started to change pretty rapidly," McDonough said. "That's really rewarding, but at the same time there are challenges. A lot of people whose careers I followed are getting pushed out of business or putting their careers on hiatus while they figure out how to adapt."

CAMBODIA: "IF YOU EAT IT, YOU WILL BE HAPPY"

Cannabis—known as *kancha* in Thailand, *kanhch* in Cambodia, and *gaj ando* in Vietnam—has a long history of use in Southeast Asia, dating to the sixth and seventh centuries when immigrants brought it over from India. For centuries, particularly in Thailand, Laos, Cambodia, and Indonesia, cannabis was used as both food and medicine, cultivated in most home gardens, and hawked by herb and spice vendors in the markets.

In Cambodia, cannabis—or ganja, based on its Indian roots—was used liberally as a seasoning in Khmer food for centuries, with no legal or moral stigma attached to it. For most Cambodians, the herb was nothing more than an ingredient in the "happy soup" that they had served at weddings and parties for generations. Then, in the 1980s, as the country began the painful process of recovering from Pol Pot's genocide in Khmer Rouge, which killed millions, backpackers from the West (that decade's hippies) arrived. Western explorers began spreading the word about Cambodia's breathtaking beaches and temples and low cost of living through their own networks and underground travel guides, and they often mentioned the country's laissez-faire attitude toward cannabis. As more and more tourists in the know began showing up in the markets in search of cannabis branches, Cambodian vendors realized the plant's value to smokers and began to offer prerolled joints alongside the stalks.

Throughout the 1980s and well into the twenty-first century, Cambodia would consistently rank among the world's most cannabis-friendly nations. In 1984, *High Times* editor Peter Gorman called Cambodia the "marijuana capital of the world" and reported that "massive amounts" of cannabis were grown there for export and tourist consumption. "With the government in transition, grass is de facto legal and sold openly in Phnom Penh markets for as little as $3 a kilo for reasonable quality," he reported.[46]

That didn't sit well with the United States, where the Reagan administration was launching its renewed drug wars and "Just Say No" campaign. In 1996, the United States put Cambodia on its list of major illicit drug-producing and drug-transit countries, largely because of its heroin trade, and forced it to pass strict antidrug laws that included marijuana. The cannabis laws were largely ignored, and many, if not most, Cambodians continued to keep a couple of plants in their culinary gardens. In a *Phnom Penh Post* article explaining Cambodia's "complicated" relationship with ganja, in which authorities make exceptions to the law for traditional and medicinal use, one cannabis farmer compared the situation to Jamaica, where cannabis was illegal but tolerated.[47]

As they had for centuries, cannabis growers continued to convene on the Mekong River during the cooler months after monsoon season to start thousands of seedlings in raised beds, sometimes alternating with corn to make the most use of limited rainwater. These growers distributed their crop to vendors in Phnom Penh and other cities, who sold them alongside yams and bitter melons as they always had. Though the newly formed antidrug police squads might come by once in a while and confiscate cannabis sellers' supplies, ganja was hardly eradicated. It remained readily available to anyone who knew how to ask.

Most Cambodians didn't smoke cannabis but used it instead to season foods like "happy soup," a basic chicken soup with cannabis, lemongrass, garlic leaf, chives, and two native mints, *chi ng yeung* and *chi bung la*, that was traditionally served in a ring dish around a small charcoal chimney.[48] As international forces pressured Cambodia to crack down on drugs, the word *happy* became code for ordering food sprinkled with cannabis in certain restaurants. In the early 1990s, the Happy Herb Pizza chain, with locations in Phnom Penh, Siem Reap, and Sihanoukville, became famous in backpacker travel guides for its practice of spreading ground cannabis on top of the tomato sauce and under the mozzarella cheese before baking their pies. "We make happy food because if you eat it, you will be happy. Everyone likes to be happy," the restaurant's advertisements said.

Happy Herb, located on a street overlooking the Tonlé Sap River near the Royal Palace in Phnom Penh, was surrounded by other restaurants such as Pink Elephant Pizza and Ecstatic Pizza that also offered "happy" pizza, and throughout the country, pizzerias and more traditional restaurants such as the Smokin' Pot in Battambang, famous for its "happy" baked chicken, offered cannabis-infused menu items. Tourists in Phnom Penh could ask their *tuk-tuk* driver to take them to a "happy" restaurant or find them clustered together, just off of the main tourist avenue. The restaurants, with or without "happy" in their name, could make anything—shakes, rice, pancakes, and of course, soup—"happy" or "extra happy" upon request.

"Happy" food was one of the worst-kept secrets on the planet. The "underground" dining experience was well-documented online in travel blogs and travel guides and in the major media. TV personality and chef Anthony Bourdain ate a "happy" pie, which he called "something of an indigenous classic around here," on his CNN show *Parts Unknown* in 2011 and dubbed it "the pizza that makes you insane in the membrane,"[49] a label that would reverberate online for years. In 2017, *Vice* "Munchies" writer Max Winkler wrote an article about eating an entire "happy" pie, "Phnom Penh's Happy Pizza Left Me High and Dry," in which he recalled, while consuming a happy coconut milkshake in Kampot, asking the restaurant owner why he opened a happy restaurant. He got a very familiar answer. "We make happy food, because if you eat it, you will be happy," the man said. "Everyone likes to be happy."[50]

INDONESIA: "ALRIGHT TO USE IT AS A FOOD SEASONING"

Cambodia's neighbor to the south, Indonesia, was also considered a hassle-free place for backpackers with Western passports to find and use cannabis well into the 1980s, even though cannabis had been illegal since Indonesia joined the 1925 International Opium Convention.

The law did little to stop farmers in the fertile Aceh region in northern Sumatra, who continued to cultivate cannabis and send it out to be sold freely from market kiosks and vegetable carts, as they always had. The Acehnese people smoked cannabis mixed with tobacco and also used it with other herbs in homemade remedies. They soaked cannabis flowers in palm wine and kept the tincture in bamboo branches to drink as a tonic and consumed cannabis and nutmeg tea to alleviate asthma, chest pain, and bile secretion. The Acehnese also used cannabis recreationally, drinking a tea made from dried cannabis leaves that induced a sense of well-being known as *hayal*, a state of imagination or fantasy.

In the kitchen, the Acehnese made use of cannabis from morning to night. They mixed it with coffee; used it to enhance flavor and moisture in goat curries, fried noodles, peanut sauce, and soups; and made a toffee-like sweet called *dodol aceh*. They ate fresh fan leaves alongside other greens and tossed them into soups and stews. Cannabis leaves were a key ingredient in *mie aceh*, a popular street food. In his cookbook about the cuisine of the Spice Islands, *Cradle of Flavor*, James Oseland wrote that cannabis provided an "earthy, green taste" to dishes such as *masam jing* (hot and sour fish stew with bamboo shoots) but noted that stinging nettles could be substituted for diners who didn't want a cannabinoid buzz.[51]

The Indonesian government began to get tough on cannabis in the late 1970s, when rebels from the separatist group Free Aceh Movement (*Gerakan Aceh Merdeka*) began funding their operations through illicit cannabis cultivation and sales. Indonesia had been under increasing international pressure to crack down on cannabis crimes since it joined the 1961 UN Single Convention on Narcotic Drugs, and in 1976, it did, with a law introducing life sentences for dealing and trafficking cannabis. In 2002, President Megawati Sukarnoputri imposed some of the world's harshest penalties, including capital punishment, for cannabis crimes. Yet the nation's cannabis users remained, for the most part, undeterred.

Nearly two million people used cannabis in Indonesia in 2014, making it the country's most used illicit substance. In Aceh, ganja continued to be a lucrative cash crop, with an expanding cottage industry of entrepreneurs finding creative ways to use the plant. One company mixed it with the region's other mainstay, coffee, to make *kopi lawak*, which means "coffee buffoonery" and is a play on *kopi luwak*, the fermented Indonesian gourmet coffee made from the excrement of civet cats. Many households continued to grow cannabis in their backyards alongside garlic and eggplant, though they often had to bribe the military not to destroy their plants. In certain restaurants throughout Aceh, diners in the know could order dishes made with ganja.

In 2007, Indonesian vice president Jusuf Kalla said cannabis should remain illegal, but "it's alright to use it as a food seasoning."[52] Indonesians and tourists who did so were certainly not without risk.

Enforcement of cannabis laws was rigorous in Indonesia. Between 2009 and 2012, as many as twenty-six people per day were imprisoned for using cannabis, and the authorities embarked on an aggressive eradication program.

In the late 2010s, the government had a slight change of heart, likely based on the number of cannabis users filling up Indonesia's prisons, and opened up discussions about legalizing medical marijuana. In 2015, *Lingkar Ganja Nusantara* (The Archipelago's Circle of Cannabis), a group founded in 2010 to inform the public about the traditional, cultural, and legal contexts of cannabis, obtained the first governmental license to conduct scientific research on the cannabis plant through its research body, *Yayasan Sativa Nusantara* (Sativa Nusantara Foundation).

BROWNIE MARY: CIVIL DISOBEDIENCE, YES; MARGARINE, NEVER

Though she had a foul mouth and her only daughter died before she had children, Mary Jane Rathbun was often described as "grandmotherly," and she knew how to use that to her advantage. The tough-talking advocate for medical marijuana, who was never afraid to break and even flout the law for her cause, was also one of the people responsible for California becoming the first state to legalize marijuana for medical use in 1996. *High Times* magazine called her a "saint." She was the Mother Teresa of cannabis.

Rathbun was certainly no saint in the conventional sense. When she was thirteen, Rathbun ran away from her conservative Catholic Minnesota family after fighting off a nun who tried to cane her. She wandered around the Midwest working as an activist for a while, taking up the causes of miners, union workers, and abortion rights before heading to San Francisco in the early 1970s. Rathbun landed in the largely gay Castro district, where she worked as a waitress in a chain restaurant and baked cannabis-infused brownies as a way to build her retirement fund. A fixture in the neighborhood, wearing her signature pantsuit and walking the streets offering rich chocolate brownies with nuts from a napkin-lined basket, Rathbun became known as Brownie Mary. Her recipe was a closely guarded secret.

Rathbun did a brisk business as word got around about her special brownies, reportedly selling about six hundred brownies at $20 per dozen, or $2 per piece, every week.[53] *High Times* reported that "almost anybody could give her a call and place an order for a batch,"[54] and customers lined up along the stairs of her apartment to wait for hours for a chance to buy a dozen or two.[55] Even so, Rathbun managed to evade the police until her hand-drawn flyers for "magically delicious" brownies, posted prominently around the neighborhood, were finally too much for them. Rathbun was arrested for the first time in 1981 and charged with eight felonies for possessing fourteen pounds of processed flour with cannabis and three ounces of psilocybin mushrooms.

Rathbun's grandmotherly presence paid off at the trial, as the judge took a shine to the fifty-seven-year-old and let her off with probation and community service. Feisty and unapologetic despite her guilty plea, with her matronly glasses and silver curls, Rathbun became a darling of the press. In an article headlined "Alice B. Toklas Goodies," the *New York Times* quipped, "The price, $20 a dozen, seemed steep even for homemade brownies, but they were selling like hot cakes, and no wonder."

When police raided her home, the *Times* reported, Rathbun said to them, "I thought you guys were coming."[56] The police alleged she was making $10,000 per week, which Rathbun neither confirmed nor denied. "Whatever I do, I'm good at," she told the *San Francisco Chronicle*, noting she could also whip up a potent pecan pie and a wicked spaghetti sauce.[57] Later, Rathbun told *High Times* she had a batch of brownies in the oven two days after she was released from jail.[58]

The volunteer work that Rathbun carried out as part of her sentence entailed shuttling patients to radiology from San Francisco General's famed Ward 86, an AIDS clinic in a converted pediatrics ward, just as the frightening new epidemic was beginning to ravage the city's gay community. She grew close with the patients, whom she called her "kids" (which contributed mightily to her grandmotherly reputation). Though Rathbun stopped selling her brownies after the arrest, she began bringing them to the ward in paper sacks and giving them to her kids to help alleviate the wasting syndrome that came with AIDS and ease the side effects of the chemotherapy they were undergoing.

"I give them away," she told *High Times*. "These kids need the medicine desperately. I want them as comfortable as possible."[59] Rathbun estimated she baked thirty-five or forty dozen brownies every three or four months, which she distributed for free to sick people all over the Bay Area during the 1980s and early 1990s. She went through hundreds of pounds of anonymously donated cannabis.[60]

In 1992, while Rathbun was making brownies at a friend's house in Sonoma County, she was arrested again, this time by the DEA and local law officials, and charged with felony possession. The narcs reported that they confiscated "35 pounds of margarine, 50 pounds of flour and sugar, 22 dozen eggs, 21,000 square feet of plastic wrap, and 20 pounds of high-grade cannabis"—in essence, offering up Rathbun's secret recipe. Worse than that for Rathbun, however, was the cops' suggestion that she used anything but the finest quality butter—she said she would never use margarine—to make her brownies.[61]

This time Rathbun refused to plead guilty, and on the day that she appeared in Municipal Court in Santa Rosa, San Francisco, supervisors declared it Brownie Mary Day in her honor. The local judge, realizing that Brownie Mary was far too beloved to prosecute, reduced the charges to misdemeanor possession, then dismissed them altogether later.

Rathbun's civil disobedience again caught the media's and the public's attention, and this time the story was picked up around the world. CNN played the Brownie Mary story heavily across its international network, airing her for-the-record quote, "I'm not going to stop baking pot brownies for my kids with AIDS!" The quote heard 'round the world was a cleaned-up version of a saltier one Rathbun offered up to several other sources. "If the narcs think I'm going to stop baking pot brownies for my kids with AIDS," she said, "they can go fuck themselves in Macy's window!"[62]

As demand for Brownie Mary's confections exploded—eventually becoming so overwhelming that Rathbun had to pull names from a cookie jar to see which AIDS patient got the next dozen—she continued to fight for her kids' right to medical marijuana. In 1993, she hooked up with her longtime friend and fellow activist Dennis Peron to found the Cannabis Buyers' Club, a five-story office space on Market Street in San Francisco that sold cannabis-infused bread, cake, brownies, "merry pills," and cannabis flowers to sick and dying AIDS and cancer patients. The club was legally possible after San Francisco voters passed a series of "compassionate use" resolutions that made enforcing cannabis laws the lowest priority for local police, and patients flocked to it like goats to new grass.

Though not the only one of its kind, the Cannabis Buyers' Club was considered the Taj Mahal of cannabis buyers' clubs, with as many as 1,700 of its 7,800 members smoking, eating, chatting, and enjoying nonalcoholic beverages in the club's three stories of lounges on any given day. Peron, who would sometimes walk through the club handing out free one-eighth-ounce bags of cannabis, joked that the club became "an auxiliary branch of the Health Department."[63] It was there that activists met to campaign for the Compassionate Use Act of 1996 to legalize medical marijuana, which was voted in as Proposition 215 in 1996.

By then, however, Rathbun was in crippling pain from arthritic knees and other ailments, reportedly eating a brownie or more a day just so she could walk, and considering assisted suicide. At Peron's urging, she hung on and lived to see her life's work come to fruition when California passed the statewide referendum.

In 1996, Rathbun and Peron published a small book about cannabis cookery, *Brownie Mary's Marijuana Cookbook and Dennis Peron's Recipe for Social Change*, which included recipes for everything from spaghetti sauce to chestnut stuffing—but not Rathbun's closely guarded secret brownie recipe, which she kept in a safe-deposit box. "When and if they legalize it, I'll sell my brownie recipe to Betty Crocker or Duncan Hines and take the profits and buy an old Victorian for my kids with AIDS," she said.[64] When she became ill, Rathbun promised to leave the recipe to Peron so he could carry out her plans, but it was never found.

Rathbun died of a heart attack at age seventy-seven on April 10, 1999, and was honored seven days later in what *High Times* described as "an old-fashioned San Francisco love-in." In his tribute, the Reverend Elder Jim Mitulski of Castro's Metropolitan Community Church declared: "Brownie Mary is stronger than death. Brownie Mary never ends."[65]

• 5 •

An Industry Is Born

The story of California's Proposition 215—which is the story of the beginning of the end of cannabis prohibition in the United States—began in 1991, when Dennis Peron and Mary Jane Rathbun led an initiative to sanction medical use of cannabis in San Francisco that passed by an overwhelming 79 percent, paving the way for the opening of the Cannabis Buyers' Club on Market Street in 1992. Peron and Rathbun took the fight to legalize medical marijuana to the California legislature and got bills passed, but Republican governor Pete Wilson vetoed them in 1994 and 1995.

Peron said he was forced to "take it to the people." In 1996, he ran the Californians for Compassionate Use campaign for Proposition 215, an initiative to legalize medical marijuana statewide, largely out of his club until a handful of major out-of-state financiers, including George Soros and Laurance Rockefeller, took over. With big money backing, the campaign won the public's heart with commercials released weeks before the election featuring cancer patients and their caregivers talking about why they were willing to break the law to relieve their loved ones' nausea and misery.

As the first statewide voter initiative to legalize cannabis in any form, Prop 215 gained national notoriety and enraged state and federal authorities. President Bill Clinton's drug czar Barry McCaffrey flew out several times before the election to meet with California's state attorney general Dan Lungren, an ambitious lawman whom local media called "Joe Friday." A senior McCaffrey aide told *Newsweek* that officials believed "every pothead in America will want to move there"[1] if the issue passed.

On October 11, 1996, Lungren authorized one hundred DEA agents armed with assault rifles and battering rams to shut down the Cannabis Buyers' Club, creating a public relations disaster for his office and the feds. Peron, led out in handcuffs, came off as a martyr, and public sympathy for the thousands of medical marijuana patients the raid sent into the streets was widespread. Lungren ended up on the wrong side of cartoonist Garry Trudeau's satire of the situation in a *Doonesbury* comic strip and called a news conference to demand that California newspapers pull the strips. Though a few reported on the news conference, none obeyed his commands.

California's Compassionate Use Act passed with 56 percent of the vote. In the same election, 65 percent of Arizona voters approved Proposition 200, giving doctors the right to prescribe medical marijuana as well as heroin and LSD and mandating treatment instead of prison terms for nonviolent drug offenders. McCaffrey, Attorney General Janet Reno, and Health and Human Services Secretary Donna Shalala called the referendums a national threat and floated a plan to discourage physicians from prescribing medical marijuana and deny tax write-offs for expenditures related to its use. McCaffrey said ad campaigns harping on compassion for the sick had "duped" voters into approving "Cheech and Chong medicine."[2]

Peron and his supporters were jubilant—in his election night speech he declared the victory "about who we are as people and where we're going as a nation"—as pundits saw cracks in the zero-tolerance drug laws that had defined the 1980s and early 1990s. "Taken together, the two initiatives mark the first popular assault on the drug war since the wave of decriminalization that swept the states in the seventies," Sarah, Duchess of York, wrote in *The Nation*.[3] *Reason* magazine declared: "'Just say no' has been answered with 'Tell us why.'"[4] Ethan Nadelmann, director of the Lindesmith Center, a policy institute promoting tolerant drug policies, said the initiatives were the first time since the repeal of Prohibition that the public had approved a pullback in the war on drugs.[5] Six more states would follow with similar initiatives in 1998.

On the day after the election, Peron reopened the Cannabis Buyers' Club. A line of patients snaked around the block, waiting to fill out paperwork that documented their diagnoses and identification so they could get newly required membership cards and partake again of joints, tinctures, and infused cookies and truffles under the origami mobiles in the club's violet-walled party room. AIDS patient Milahhr Kemnah purchased two $5 bags of low-grade Mexican flowers and became the first person since the 1930s to buy cannabis under state law protection.[6]

Soon more than thirty cannabis clubs, which Lester Grinspoon described as "a blend of Amsterdam-style coffeehouse, American bar, and support group,"[7] had opened in the area. The clubs were nothing if not open-minded in admission standards, as Michael Pollan revealed in the *New York Times* the next year. At the Cannabis Buyers' Club, Pollan watched an MS patient, "pretzeled into his wheelchair, his arms and hands too badly bent to sign his name to the application form," get a membership card with a letter from a social worker rather than a doctor, as required, because the intake staffer was too compassionate to turn him away. "What I was witnessing here was something other than medicine—it was, in fact, a lot closer to religion. Peron is California's evangelist of marijuana, and he has drawn around him a following—people sick in body or soul—who come to his church, many of them daily."[8]

Two months after the election, in a case backed by Lungren, US prosecutors sought permanent injunctions against the Cannabis Buyers' Club and five others for selling cannabis in violation of federal law. They were fighting a losing battle, as medical marijuana had already flowered into an ask-permission-later industry of growers and distributors operating under a law that officials had little or no understanding of nor consensus about how to implement.

Peron quietly pleaded guilty to being a public nuisance, a misdemeanor, and was given time served for an earlier incarceration in 2001 as public sentiment and the political climate in California turned in medical marijuana's favor. Lungren's replacement as attorney general had no interest in pursuing felonies against the white-haired activist whom thousands of people considered a saint. Peron married his longtime partner when same-sex marriage became legal, and he died of lung cancer at his home and former bed-and-breakfast, Castro Castle, in 2018.

Meanwhile, medical marijuana became an industry. In 2003, Democratic governor Gray Davis signed Senate Bill 420, establishing ID cards for medical marijuana patients and allowing patients to pay "reasonable compensation" to primary caregivers or "collectives" for services that enabled them to use medical marijuana. That was all the encouragement eager ganjapreneurs in California needed. Cannabis clubs like Peron's and nonprofit patient collectives morphed into chains of retail stores supported by a network of hydroponics suppliers, physicians, lawyers, public relations and real estate specialists, chefs, and other professionals.

Local jurisdictions were allowed to amend the state guidelines, and the nascent industry was far more welcome in some cities than others, leading to oversaturation in cities like Oakland—a city that dealt with constant budget shortfalls and debt, it was among the first and most vocal of the municipalities to welcome the industry, declaring itself the Silicon Valley of Weed—and vast swaths of medical marijuana deserts in places like Orange County. "The limited legal protections afforded to pot growers and dispensary owners have turned marijuana cultivation and distribution in California into a classic 'gray area' business, like gambling or strip clubs, which are tolerated or not, to varying degrees, depending on where you live and on how aggressive your sheriff is feeling that afternoon," David Samuels reported in *The New Yorker* in 2008.

Samuels described "collectives" like The Farmacy, a high-end boutique with stores in West Hollywood, Venice, and Westwood, that offered cannabis-infused herbal gelato and a bamboo-bound menu, kept behind the counter, describing cannabis strains that could be had for a $75 per gram "donation," along with a selection of Chinese herbs, Asian handicrafts, and organic soaps.[9] By 2010, the State Board of Equalization estimated medical marijuana dispensaries were producing $1.3 billion in over-the-counter transactions and $100 million in state sales taxes.[10]

The California cannabis market showed no signs of stopping, and the sky appeared to be the limit. In the 2012 finale of *Weeds*, Showtime's eight-season series about Nancy Botwin, an upper-middle-class mom in a fictional Los Angeles suburb who started out dealing cannabis to survive after her husband died and ended up in a series of adventures including gangs and drug lords, Nancy sold her chain of fifty cannabis cafés called Good Seed to Starbucks. The show was futuristic, but not so far off.

In 2006, Steve DeAngelo, an entrepreneur and longtime cannabis advocate immediately recognizable by his fedora and long braids, opened what he called the world's largest medical marijuana dispensary promoting cannabis as a "wellness" drug for healthy everyday living. The glistening glass cases at his seven-thousand-square-foot store between the 880 Freeway and Oakland's industrial waterfront offered more than five dozen cannabis strains, elixirs, creams, lotions, and chewy chocolate edibles with hash frosting in addition to acupuncture, chiropractic, and life coaching sessions and yoga. Harborside had more than fifty thousand registered medical marijuana patients and served more than eight hundred of them per day, bringing in more than $20 million and paying more than $2.3 million in state taxes and fees by 2010. Two years later, more than 100,000 patients joined a San Jose outlet.[11]

COLORADO: "HOW DO WE GET A PIECE?"

When the seeds of reefer madness were being planted in the United States at the turn of the twentieth century, Colorado—where racism against Mexican immigrants was institutional and rampant—was one of the first states to jump on board. The state made use and cultivation of cannabis a misdemeanor in 1917. Then in 1929, the Colorado legislature reacted swiftly to a sensationalized murder involving a Mexican immigrant and made cannabis use and cultivation a felony. It remained that way until 1975, when the Colorado legislature followed a briefly lived national trend and decriminalized possession, transportation, and private use of up to an ounce of cannabis, making it a petty offense with a maximum fine of $100.

In 2000, two years after California voted in medical marijuana, Colorado voters approved Amendment 20, allowing the use and cultivation of medical marijuana. A handful of dispensaries immediately cropped up in Denver's sketchier neighborhoods to meet the needs of registered medical marijuana patients (and sometimes others), but the Colorado marketplace didn't really get underway until 2007, when Denver district judge Larry Naves ruled that caregivers could grow plants for an unlimited number of patients. Dispensaries fought for patient "members" who would declare them their "caregiver," allowing the dispensary to grow their physician-allotted number of plants—anywhere from six to hundreds—in mega grows housed in homes and warehouses around the state.

In 2009, US Deputy Attorney General David W. Ogden released a memo declaring the federal government would not go after patients who used cannabis for cancer or other serious illnesses or their caregivers, as long as they were in clear and unambiguous compliance with existing state law, and told US attorneys to consider enforcing cannabis laws as their lowest priority. Most people in the Colorado cannabis industry, and elsewhere, interpreted the memo as permission to conduct cannabis commerce without fear of federal prosecution, and that was all the odd mix of outlaw growers and brazen businesspeople who had been circling the quasi-legal new industry needed.

"That's when the floodgates opened," said cannabis activist Mason Tvert, founder of Safer Alternative for Enjoyable Recreation.[12] The Green Rush was on. In cities that allowed them, dispensaries were on every corner, as prominent as Starbucks. Upscale boutiques and spa-like "wellness" centers that also offered acupuncture and massage began to edge out the basement speakeasies with green neon cannabis leaves in their barred windows that had pioneered the market. The alternative newspaper *Westword* added a weekly advice column, "Ask a Stoner."

The industry was a far cry from the buttoned-up billion-dollar business it would become in those early days. Jeanna Hoch, who ran a Denver dispensary, Medicinal Alternatives, and an edible company, Mile High Metamunchies, from 2008 to 2009, remembers an industry run by "a lot of shady players." As "front desk girl" for the dispensary, she said, "I did all the files, made sure everything looked dispensary-ish. And we're like, what does that look like? What is a dispensary? We've never really seen one. We've never been in one."

Medicinal Alternatives was registered with the Colorado Secretary of State, and that was all Hoch and her team knew to do as far as legalities went. They wanted to play by the rules, but they had trouble figuring out what the rules actually were. "It was pertinent to all of us to figure out how to get into the legal side of it," Hoch said, "but it was also really important to us because we had worked so hard in the illegal aspect. It was like this was our industry. This is who we are, what we've done. We are the growers. We are the salesmen. We are the consumers. This is where we should be. Colorado is opening it up. How do we get a piece?"[13]

"Underground," is how Wanda James, an entrepreneur and politician who was the first African American woman to own a medical marijuana dispensary in Colorado, remembered the scene when she opened Apothecary of Colorado with her husband, chef and restaurateur Scott Durrah, in 2009. "Everybody wanted to keep their head down, and not talk about it. This was still a lot of the people that were coming from the underground marijuana movement, moving into owning the businesses," James said. "So many people were fearful, and they were fearful of even the people like myself, that wanted to bring attention to it."

When James and Durrah opened their dispensary in Denver's hip city center Highlands neighborhood just west of I-25, where high-rise condos and loft buildings were just beginning to replace the neighborhood's older single-story buildings, people thought they were crazy. The power couple owned a popular downtown Jamaican restaurant, 8 Rivers. James, who had deep political connections through her consulting firm James Foxx, had served on the national finance committee for President Obama and run a successful campaign for Congressman Jared Polis. Their friend, a *Denver Post* columnist, warned them that people would shun them and stop eating at 8 Rivers.

The couple, who were both passionate about cannabis legalization and not afraid to speak out for the plant they believed in, were undeterred. "I'm black, hello," Durrah said. "The bottom line is, it's a social justice issue. My brother-in-law Rick was arrested with two ounces of weed on him and given seven years in the penitentiary in Texas, picking cotton." Durrah paused. "A black man, picking cotton in the South. In the '90s."

Aware that she was a moving target, James "minimized the risk to the nth degree," keeping two senators and one congressman on speed dial. She was caught up in a movement with deep social implications that mattered to her as an African American, a woman, and a cannabis consumer. "Clearly, too, it was the time," James said. "I think with any movement, or any leadership piece that comes from people or masses, it's because of a time and a movement. Martin Luther King wouldn't have worked in the '30s. Each time we find the right time for a movement, and this was our time. Our collective time."

The first obstacle James and Durrah had to deal with was the public's perception that Apothecary of Colorado's five hundred registered patients were all twenty-one-year-old snowboarders with mohawks, scoring recreational drugs based on bogus prescriptions for "chronic pain." That could not have been farther from the truth, James said. "They were forty-year-old women experiencing severe pain from breast cancer. They were sixty-five-year-old women going through menopausal-type issues. They were older men with stomach cancer. They were thirty-five-year-old guys with arthritis in the knees."

One of those patients, an eighty-five-year-old man with a grapefruit-sized tumor, inspired Durrah to take his culinary experiments with cannabis-infused food to the next level. The man told Durrah he wanted to have dinner with his wife one last time, without morphine. "I lost it," Durrah said. "What that told me at that moment was that whatever I was doing, this was the connection to a man's life. Everything came from that moment for my wife and me." Durrah began offering cooking classes on Saturday mornings at 8 Rivers, consistently packing the room to capacity with seventy-five or more students. "It was unbelievable how many people wanted these classes," James said.

In Colorado, a cottage industry of edibles, mostly baked goods whipped up in home kitchens and distributed in plastic wrap packaging, was just getting started. Chefs would bring their brownies or cookies to Apothecary of Colorado, James recalled, and if she and Durrah liked them, they would buy them to stock their shelves. Appalled at the lack of standards and regulatory oversight for everything from potency to kitchen sanitation, the couple dove into the edibles industry, determined to bring a level of professionalism that didn't yet exist.

They sold Apothecary of Colorado in 2010 and opened Simply Pure Medicated Edibles, offering a diverse line of organic, vegan, gluten-free edibles that included coconut almond cups, sesame brittle, marinara sauce, mango salsa, and peanut butter, all made with food-grade hash and cannabis-infused coconut oil. They set up a professional kitchen and a ten-thousand-square-foot facility to grow cannabis organically and hired four professional chefs, a taste engineer who had worked at Hershey, and fifteen salespeople across the state. Simply Pure was the first edibles company in Colorado to offer something other than candy and baked goods. "Scott was now cooking for people at end of life," James said. "There are only so many brownies a sick person can eat."

By 2010, state officials realized they needed to take control of this industry that had grown into a wild, wild west, with nothing more than a patchwork of poorly understood local regulations to oversee it. The Colorado Legislature responded by passing House Bill 1284, creating the world's first system to regulate and tax for-profit cannabis businesses, requiring dispensary owners to register with the state, pass criminal background checks, install security systems, pay taxes, grow 70 percent of their own product, and meticulously track their inventory from seed to sale.

The regulations shook out a lot of smaller players who didn't have the resources to do the paperwork and pay for security and tracking systems, and they escalated industry consolidation that would only get more intense as larger manufacturers flooded the market with less expensive edibles.

EDIBLES IN COLORADO: "HOCKEY-STICK GROWTH"

On election night in 2012, Mason Tvert, a key figure in the passage of Amendment 64, which legalized adult use of cannabis, stayed up all night and into the next morning doing press interviews and news shows, as media outlets around the world ran with the story about the first state to legalize adult use of cannabis. (Washington State voters also approved cannabis legalization, but an hour after Colorado.) At an 11 a.m. press conference in front of the Capitol, Tvert looked around at the hundred or so reporters and said, "We called this press conference to find out where all of you people have been for our previous press conferences."[14]

Perhaps no one was more amazed than the people who made it happen when 55 percent of Colorado voters approved Amendment 64 on November 6, 2012. That night, an ecstatic crowd of Amendment 64 volunteers and supporters packed into the dance hall at Casselman's, a bar and music venue in Denver's RiNo district, cheering, crying, hugging, and high-fiving when the results were announced. "It was just this packed house of people that had supported us over the years and then people that had driven in from out of town that just wanted to see what it would be like if marijuana became legal. People that had spent years and decades of their lives in prison for marijuana were in that room," said attorney Brian Vicente, who along with his partner, Christian Sederberg, was instrumental in getting Amendment 64 passed.[15]

With much fanfare, the first legal cannabis sale took place in Denver on January 1, 2013. Lines snaked down city blocks to buy flowers, edibles, and concentrates in the new retail stores. Sales were immediately robust, with demand for edibles exceeding all expectations. In the first year, $700 million worth of medical and recreational cannabis—seventy-five tons of flower and fifty million edibles—was sold in Colorado.[16]

When edibles sales tripled in 2014,[17] issues that had been plaguing the industry—inconsistent dosing, overconsumption, accidental ingestion, and pesticide residues—could no longer be ignored. In June 2014, *New York Times* columnist Maureen Dowd wrote an infamous column, "Don't Harsh Our Mellow, Dude,"[18] about a bad trip she had after eating an innocent-looking caramel-chocolate candy bar from a cannabis store in Denver. The people who hosted Dowd on a bus tour of Denver's cannabis scene claimed they told her that Colorado's recommended dose of THC was ten milligrams and that each little square of the chocolate bar she bought at a retail dispensary was one dose. But Dowd got impatient and either forgot or ignored the advice she'd been given and ate more. While she was waiting for the effects to come on, she drank some chardonnay.

Dowd's resulting freakout became cannabis legend. Her column not only chronicled the overdose in horrifying detail but also noted that a nineteen-year-old college student had jumped off a Denver hotel balcony after eating a cookie with sixty-five milligrams of THC and a Denver man had killed his wife after eating cannabis-infused Karma Kandy. It was just one in a string of bad publicity hits, including reports of more children accidentally overdosing, that resulted in national scrutiny of the burgeoning edibles industry—and also led to some hilarious new phrases for overconsuming such as "overdowding" and "dowd and out."

State regulators again stepped in, enacting measures that required childproof packaging, ten-milligram-per-serving dosing size restrictions, a universal THC symbol stamped onto every serving, and contamination and potency testing information. The new regulations shook out another round of smaller players, who couldn't afford the packaging or keep up with the paperwork. "It was a challenge for everybody," said Nancy Whiteman, a former insurance executive who founded Wana, one of Colorado's most successful candy businesses, in 2010 (see photo on next page). "We had to relook at formulation of some of our products. We had this really delicious caramel, but it was so buttery that it wouldn't hold a stamp. What doesn't kill you makes you stronger, right?"

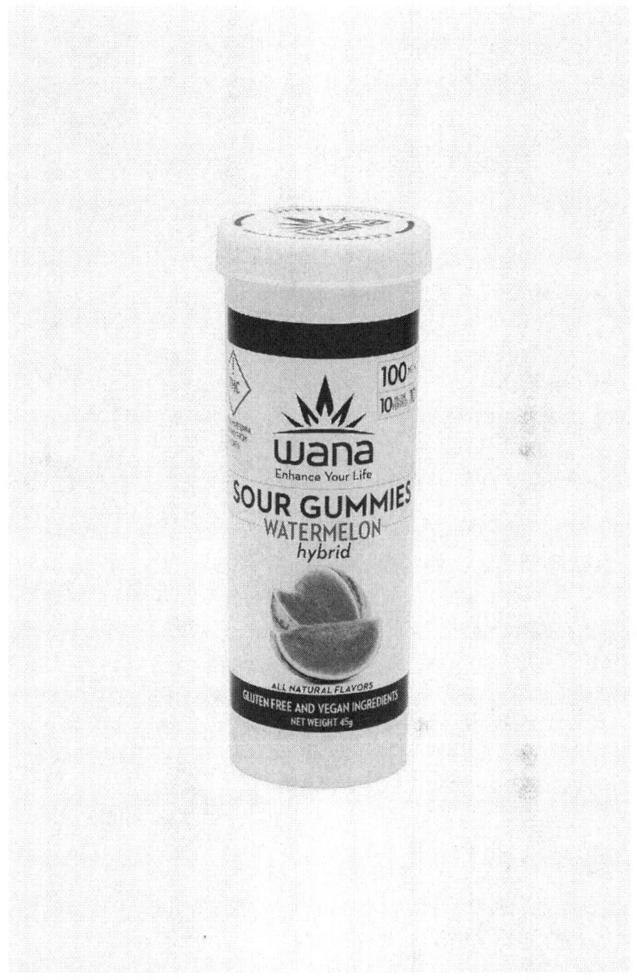

Wana gummies were one of the most popular cannabis-infused candies in Colorado.

The major players who were left to rule the market smelled money. In an interview with *Rolling Stone* just as Colorado's adult-use market was opening up in 2014, Tripp Keber, who founded Dixie Elixirs & Edibles, one of Colorado's largest manufacturers of THC-infused soda, candy, and baked goods for the medical marijuana

The Art of Extraction

As soon as humans figured out that the cannabis plant's magic was in the sticky resin on its inner leaves and flowers, they began improving on nature. After they rubbed the flowers with their fingers, and eventually a sieve, to separate out these crystals (*kief*), they pressed them into concentrated wafers or blocks—the first *hashish.* Some variation of this basic technique was used throughout the ages, until the intersection of legalization and technology pushed the art to new levels.

Modern extraction artists used some type of solvent, CO_2, or dry ice to extract cannabinoid-rich resin glands from the plant matter to make highly concentrated extracts with 80 percent or more THC or CBD. These concentrates were easier to work with than cannabis flowers and imparted less herbal flavor because the plant material had been removed, and they were more widely used than flower in both industrial and home kitchens by the 2010s.

"Hash and concentrates are incredible culinary ingredients that taste better than flower," said Elise McDonough, a writer and cannabis industry consultant. "We'll see everything go that way. We'll be using kief as a seasoning."

Kief: The simplest of all concentrates, kief is concentrated trichomes separated from the plant when plant matter is sieved through a screen or extracted using dry ice and bubble bags. Kief can be pressed into rigid wafers.
Hash: Compressed resin from mature female cannabis flowers has been known for centuries as *hashisch* or hash, which ethnobotanist Chris Kilham called "the cognac of ganja products."
Hash Oil: Resinous oil is squeezed from the plant using pressure, temperature, or solvents.
Bubble Hash: Cannabis plant material is vigorously blended with ice and water to separate resin, which is dried and cured.
Butane Hash Oil: Butane is used to extract cannabinoids and terpenes, creating a crumbly, doughlike mixture ("budder"), a honeycomblike substance ("wax"), or a glassy, taffylike substance ("shatter").
Distillate: Concentrating, extracting, and isolating cannabinoids and terpenes from the cannabis plant via steam or franctionation, resulting in a liquid product.
Full Melt Hash: Solvents such as butane, CO_2, ether, and oxygen create a soft, waxy concentrate that melts easily when heated.
Tincture: Liquid concentrates extracted through alcohol, which capture all the cannabinoids and terpenes, were the primary means of cannabis delivery until the plant was outlawed in 1937. They can also be made with vegetable glycerin.

market, was unabashedly optimistic about the industry's future, suggesting it was about to see "hockey-stick growth." Keber said Wall Street analysts were predicting the industry would mint two or three billionaires in the next ten years. "I'm not saying I'm going to be one of them," he said, "but this kind of opportunity comes around only once in a generation."[19]

By 2017, sales of flower, edibles, and concentrates hit $1.51 billion in Colorado, delivering more than $247 million in taxes and fees to the state's coffers,[20] but breaking into the cannabis industry would not be easy for anyone. Companies like Dixie Elixirs had the market cornered, and the more the legal cannabis market matured, the further the edibles industry consolidated. By 2018, just five top brands accounted for half of all edibles sales, the top ten brands for more than two-thirds, and the top twenty for almost 90 percent, according to BDS Analytics.[21]

"The momentum is with cannabis, and it's going to take a lot of effort to derail that. It's just not slowing down," said Whiteman. "We're at the end of the first inning. It's so early in terms of what we're going to know about the plant and how to use it effectively, how to extract and recombine it. There's so much more power to this plant than what we are able to access today."

THREE COLORADO CHOCOLATE COMPANIES

Colorado was a magnet for entrepreneurs willing to take a risk when the edibles market detonated in the 2010s. Most of them didn't survive, but a handful of chocolate makers did, and they dominated the market.

Derek Cumings was inspired to become an extraction artist after he paid $80 for his first legal pan of Betty Crocker pot-butter brownies, in a red-and-white-checkered cardboard container swathed in plastic wrap, at a Denver-area dispensary not long after Colorado voters legalized medical marijuana in 2000. He and a friend devoured the entire pan while sitting in the dispensary's barbed-wire-enclosed parking lot, then waited, waited some more, and . . . nothing. The nonevent launched Cumings's quest for the holy grail of effective, reliably dosed cannabis delivery.

In 2010, he joined Bob Eschino and Rick Scarpello as a codirector of Medically Correct, Colorado's largest cannabis-infused food producer. Scarpello, who invented Udi's gluten-free bread, and Eschino, a veteran in the food packaging and marketing industry, were making and distributing cannabis-infused baked goods with a chef handpicked from Udi's—and no reliable means of getting cannabis into the brownies. "We knew we needed to become an extraction company," Scarpello said, "and we sought out Derek."

Cumings convinced the partners to invest in closed-loop butane extraction equipment, which nearly bankrupt the company but allowed it to consistently produce the concentrated THC oil it needed as it transitioned to making chocolate bars, which were less bulky, easier to consistently dose, and had a much longer shelf life than baked goods. Incredibles, a beloved line of chocolate bars in Colorado, was born.

Medically Correct officially became an extraction company with Incredibles Extracts and Extractors in 2014 and began licensing operations for Incredibles chocolates and extractions in other states. In 2017, Medically Correct employed eighty people and ran three grows with 2,300 plants, a ten-thousand-square-foot production facility, and the country's first Class 1 Division 1 ETL-certified lab for closed-loop butane cannabinoid and terpene extractions out of two warehouses in west Denver.[22]

In 2010, Andrew Schrot, fresh out of college, moved from Florida to Denver with an $80,000 loan from his parents, intent on creating an edibles company. While he and a friend were researching the market, his friend ate a cookie with a label that said it had one hundred milligrams of THC but that a budtender said had tested at fifty. After all the edibles they'd eaten during their research, the friends figured they had tolerance; fifty to one hundred milligrams didn't seem insanely high. When Schrot's friend passed out for sixteen hours, Schrot didn't know what to do. "The whole dosing thing wasn't really talked about back then," he said.

The experience made Schrot hyperconscious about dosing. He launched his company, BlueKudu, in 2011 with a tempered chocolate roll that got rave reviews from dispensary patients but was cumbersome to cut into accurately dosed pieces. A year later, BlueKudu switched gears and started making ten-piece chocolate bars that were easily breakable into squares with ten milligrams of THC each because Schrot knew dosing would become a huge factor in the growth and acceptance of edibles in Colorado.

His products were a hit, but Schrot, like everyone in the industry, struggled with constantly changing regulations and lack of access to banks and tax write-offs because the federal government still considered cannabis illegal. "In this business, half the battle, if not more, is remaining compliant," Schrot said. "And it's so expensive to remain compliant, especially when we can't have tax write-offs or get reasonable loans."

In 2017, BlueKudu moved into an 8,400-square-foot warehouse in northeast Denver with a six-figure explosion-proof extraction room that turned 150 pounds of cannabis trim into concentrate mixed with four thousand pounds of Rainforest Alliance and Fair Trade–certified artisan chocolate in a clean, spacious kitchen that produced forty-five thousand chocolate bars every month.[23]

Seeing opportunity in low-dose chocolates, former Morgan Stanley director Peter Barsoom left New York City for Colorado with his partner, Ghita Tarzi, in 2015 to build a company based on the idea that "most of us don't have six hours to have a date with an edible."

Barsoom sought to formulate products that would deliver reliable "moods and experiences" without getting people "blasted." His company, 1906—named for the year Congress enacted the Pure Food and Drug Act, which paved the way for and effectively launched cannabis prohibition—had a mission of bringing consumers back to pre-Prohibition days, when people could reliably dose themselves with over-the-counter elixirs made from cannabis and other herbs.

In November 2016, 1906 hit the shelves of about fifteen Colorado dispensaries with premium boxed chocolates marrying cacao, cannabis, and other ethnobotanical ingredients like corydalis (used in Traditional Chinese Medicine to treat insomnia) and theobromine (a stimulant already found in chocolate) in three strain-specific "experiences": Go, with Whiteout, theobromine, caffeine, theanine, and yohimbe for body energy; Pause, with Pokie and magnolia for calm; and Midnight, with Blue Dream and corydalis for sleep. High Love, with Blue Dream, damiana, muira puama, catuaba, yohimbe, and theobromine for romance, was released later.

Barsoom claimed the chocolates, with five milligrams of THC each, took effect more quickly than other edibles because of technology formulated by 1906 chief scientist Justin Kirkland, who spent years developing drug-delivery techniques for the pharmaceutical industry, which encapsulated cannabinoid molecules with lipids (fats) that protected them from being destroyed in the large intestine, pushing them into the small intestine and bloodstream more quickly.

The goal was to bring together nature (organically grown cannabis and plant medicines) and science (faster delivery, consistency, and dosing) to offer "an elevated cannabis experience," Barsoom said. "We set out to create a line of products for health-conscious adults focused on experiences that had great flavor and were fast acting. We started with chocolate because chocolate is universally loved and there's science behind how cannabis and chocolate both affect the endocannabinoid system. It's a great medium."[24]

TURNING ON TO TERPENES

From the time cannabis concentrates were invented, the extraction artists who made them were engaged in a mad race to elevate and enhance the presence of THC (and later, CBD), largely ignoring and often destroying the plant's valuable terpenes in the process. In the late 2010s, as law reforms began to unravel the research restrictions that had been a noose around scientists' necks throughout Prohibition, researchers began to prove terpenes' value as mood, taste, and health enhancers—and companies rushed in to capture and capitalize.

"The actual body of knowledge about cannabis terpenes is very small," said Ben Cassiday, cofounder of Oregon-based True Terpenes, a company that sold food-grade, strain-specific terpene formulas from noncannabis feedstock to be used in making concentrates, edibles, and topicals. "We've been repackaging and citing the same papers by Dr. [Ethan] Russo for years. I think we're going to see an emergence of new researchers producing really good work as well as anecdotal results and consumers taking it upon themselves to identify which terpenes they enjoy and don't enjoy."

Cannabis chefs discovered terpenes and used them to enhance food's taste and effects and give their creations an otherworldly zest. "Terpenes add a flavor I've never experienced in twenty-five years of cooking," said cannabis chef Randy Placeres of Aspen Culinary Solutions. "They're going to change the culinary dynamic of cuisine and chefs all over the world."[25]

In both wholesale and retail markets in legal states and countries, extracted and distilled terpenes, from both cannabis plants and noncannabis plants, were the new black. Dispensaries and retail stores offered everything from terpene concentrates and vaping liquids to terpene cooking oils. Terpene-enhanced beer and spirits became all the rage as brewers and distillers gave their products a dank edge by adding pinene and myrcene. Heineken-owned Lagunitas Brewing and CannaCraft's AbsoluteXtracts joined forces to create SuperCritical, a grassy terpene ale available only in California.

In Colorado, a company that sold postharvest management systems to growers and extractors took a Dr. Frankenstein approach, mapping different strains' naturally occurring terpene profiles through granular testing, then recreating and enhancing them with terpenes from noncannabis plants for enhancements that could be applied to cannabis flowers and concentrates. "We can create flavor and aroma combinations henceforth unknown," said Joe Edwards, head of the terpene development program at Yofumo, "and that's where we're pushing the technology."

Dr. Brian Reid, chief scientist at Colorado-based Ebbu, spent years proving that terpenes could increase THC's potency and reduce anxiety as he formulated Ebbu's vape oils and water-soluble drops engineered to deliver a consistent, predictable user experience every time. Reid said his team could demonstrate that "beyond just the wonderful aroma effects, terpenes do have specific pharmacology."

"Brian has proven scientifically and qualitatively, through cell lines and cell studies and quantifiable data, that the entourage effect does exist," said Dr. Andrew Chadeayne, Ebbu's vice president of innovation. "Terpenes are psychoactive and synergistic. They modulate cannabinoids. That's extraordinary."

WATER SOLUBILITY: A GAME CHANGER

For centuries, cannabis cooks throughout the world relied on the same basic techniques for extracting fat-soluble cannabinoids and terpenes from the plant. They would slowly simmer flowers and leaves in something oleaginous (butter, oil, cream) or macerate them in a spirit (gin, vodka, everclear) to extract the terpenes and cannabinoids (THC and CBD, primarily). These methods, time tested as they were, were far from perfect.

For one thing, lipids are one of the least efficient ways to deliver cannabinoids and terpenes to the blood, which is about 80 percent water, and fats are tough to homogenize throughout a recipe—which is crucially important for equal distribution of THC. For another, the methods left people on raw, low-fat, or alcohol-free diets without many options. And finally (and perhaps most importantly), THC and CBD were less bioavailable and took longer to come on, with potentially more potent and unpredictable effects, when processed through the liver.

Then in the 2010s came the invention of water-soluble cannabinoids and terpenes, available in powders and liquids that could be folded into any dish or beverage just like vanilla or salt, making it possible for cooks to easily stir reliable doses of cannabinoids and terpenes into any food or beverage. The innovation shook up the cannabis food scene as considerably as TV dinners and cake mixes revolutionized home cooking in the mid-twentieth century.

Naturally Splendid USA claimed the first USPTO patent for water-soluble cannabinoids, which were essential to its hemp-based Natera nutraceuticals, in 2014. In the years following, several cannabis companies won or sought patents that tweaked the process of emulsifying cannabinoids into nano-size particles that dissolved into water and mixed more easily into blood.

Juan Ayala, chief technology officer for Seattle-based Tarukino, said his company invested heavily in Sorse—emulsion technology that allows it to manufacture water-soluble cannabis liquids and powders for the wholesale market and consumer products such as Happy Apple and Utopia sparkling water—because it believed water-soluble cannabinoids were the cannabis industry's future. The company's scientists worked for more than two years to break cannabinoids and terpenes into ever-tinier particles for maximum absorption while removing or improving their bitter taste.

With its drink line, Tarukino targeted soccer moms, who could just as easily and discreetly sip a Utopia sparkling water as they could a LaCroix. The company went after home cooks with its Pro 20 and Pro-Mini cannabis-infused water sold in bottles with dosing cups. The biggest hurdle, Ayala said, was getting people to understand how simple the product was to use. "People are having a really hard time understanding it's just water," he said. "You can make pancakes, soup, ramen, guacamole . . . anything. The only dishes you can't make are ones in which you throw away the water, like spaghetti."[26]

Colorado-based Stillwater Brands ran into similar issues when it started marketing Ripple cold-water soluble powders derived from distillate, said brand director Missy Bradley. The team had to explain again and again to people who thought Ripple was a sugar packet that the powder was tasteless, odorless, calorie-free, and could be stirred into anything (see photo below). Stillwater's lead food scientist Keith Woelfel, who left Mars, Inc., to join the startup in 2016, said his team "spent considerable time and gone to great lengths to achieve consistency in dosing and clean, consistent flavor without green, hashy bitterness."

In 2017, Jon Cooper, founder and CEO of Colorado-based Ebbu, which sold liquid cannabinoid formulations engineered to produce certain moods to the wholesale and consumer markets, predicted water-soluble technology would create seismic shifts in the food and alcohol world in the next five years. "Our most important message as we move

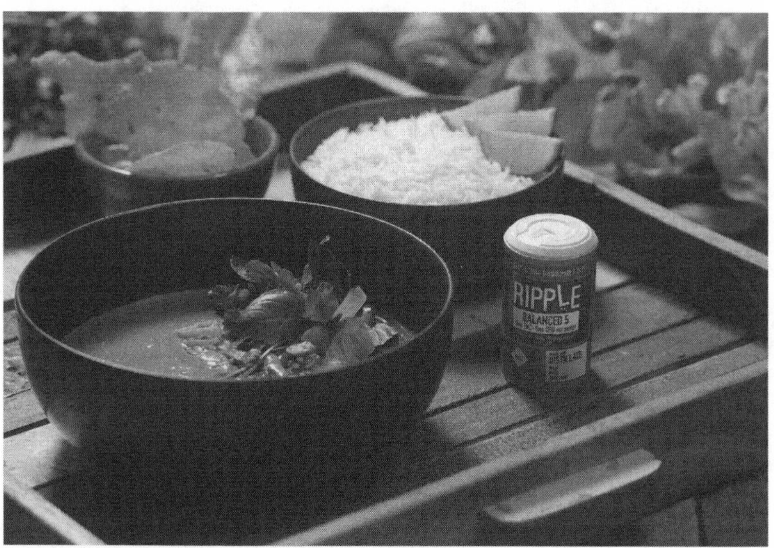

Stillwater's water-soluble powder can be added to any dish. Photo by Chad Chisholm/Courtesy of Stillwater.

forward as an industry is trust, control, responsibility and safety," Cooper said. "People will never trust products that don't deliver consistent experiences. Big companies coming into this space will have no choice but to achieve that."[27]

CHALLENGES IN COLORADO: "OVERDOWDING" AND THE "GUMMY BEAR PROBLEM"

No one thought it would be easy. Creating the world's first system to regulate and tax a substance that had been illegal for adults to use for eighty years—and remained so in the rest of the world—was a gargantuan task. And of all the challenges that undertaking entailed, said the man tasked with implementing retail sales in Colorado, edibles were the biggest.

"When we rolled out the regulation of retail edibles, we mirrored it very much after medical marijuana," Ron Kammerzell, senior director of enforcement at Colorado Department of Revenue, told *Al Jazeera* in 2015, a year after his state's voters made adult use of cannabis legal. "The thing we didn't anticipate is that the average consumer for medical marijuana is extremely knowledgeable about the effects of THC, the effects of how edible products interact with their bodies. We really didn't anticipate we'd have the challenges with possible overconsumption of edibles on the recreational market."[28]

When a delegation from Vermont visited Colorado to learn more about legalized cannabis in 2015, the challenges with edibles were the most talked-about issues they encountered. In their report about the exploratory trip, the Vermont officials observed that the problems included "marketing attractive snacks of uncertain dosage to consumers who are often naïve" and "THC candies and cookies that closely resemble non-THC candy and cookies, leading to accidental ingestions by children"—commonly referred to as the "gummy bear problem."[29]

Parents' groups and state regulators were concerned that too many cannabis-infused edibles looked too much like regular food, and in 2014, the Hershey Company sued an edibles manufacturer for infringing its Almond Joy trademark with a candy bar called Ganja Joy. "While some companies are making mandarin-flavored sodas and rich dark-chocolate bars infused with the drug, advocates for tighter marijuana regulation say that others are simply coating brightly colored bulk candy and child-friendly breakfast cereals with cannabis oil and selling it at a huge markup," the *New York Times* reported in 2014. "And critics argue that even seasoned marijuana consumers are getting sick or losing control after eating marijuana snacks that proved far more potent than they had realized. A single candy bar or soda could be packed with enough THC . . . to serve ten people."[30]

Maureen Dowd's column heard round the world was just the beginning. An increase in emergency room visits by people who had eaten too much cannabis-infused food and children who had accidentally ingested edibles made headlines. Across the country, in states that were bringing on medical marijuana programs or decriminalizing cannabis, the National Poison Data System reported increases in the number of unintentional exposure cases in young children and cannabis-related calls to poison control centers. In Aurora, Colorado, a study found that out-of-town patient visits for THC overdose increased significantly, which the study's authors attributed to the higher potency of industrially cultivated cannabis and tourists' lack of familiarity with edibles.[31]

The problem became a crisis, leaving industry leaders, regulators, and state lawmakers scrambling. No one had seen it coming. Up until that time, even after Colorado House Bill 1284 created a medical marijuana state licensing authority in 2010, no one had been paying much attention to food safety and standards. The Marijuana Enforcement Division, under the Department of Revenue, focused on law enforcement and tracking the plant, leaving no one to regulate processing and safety standards for edibles. Cannabis-infused food products weren't tested for potency, and dosing and food safety standards were wildly inconsistent.

After the public messes of 2014, things changed. The Marijuana Inventory Tracking System was implemented to follow every single cannabis plant grown in Colorado from seed to sale. (Designed to keep legally grown plants out of the black market, MITS also made it possible to track issues such as pesticide contamination and salmonella outbreaks to their source.) Edibles sold in adult-use stores were required to be wrapped or demarked in segments containing ten milligrams or less of activated THC and stamped with the letters *THC* and an exclamation point. Gummies could not be shaped like animals, fruits, or people.

Some of the bigger issues with overconsumption of edibles could be effectively addressed only through consumer education. Perhaps the most common problem was people thinking edibles were not working because of their delayed onset and eating more while they were waiting to get high ("overdowding"). The resulting overdose, which could last for twenty-four hours or more, could induce anxiety attacks and psychotic-like symptoms, the *New England Journal of Medicine* reported in 2015. "Literature regarding such cases of 'cannabis-induced psychosis' is limited, but the condition is believed to be the result of overconsumption of THC, and many of the reported cases occur following ingestion of an edible," the journal stated.[32]

Because many consumers also didn't understand that cannabis affected them differently and lasted longer when it was eaten rather than smoked—Colorado's Department of Revenue found that one milligram of THC in edibles produced behavioral effects similar to 5.71 milligrams of smoked cannabis[33]—the state, industry groups, and individual businesses launched campaigns urging cannabis consumers to "start low and go slow" as well as education platforms designed for the budtenders who sold the edibles.

These campaigns, combined with the beefed-up state regulation and oversight, helped put out some of the fires raging around the edibles markets, in Colorado and beyond. Still, when Massachusetts officials met with Colorado officials to learn more about what they were in for just weeks before that state's voters legalized adult use in 2016, Colorado director of marijuana coordination Andrew Freedman was less than encouraging about edibles. Allowing edibles to be sold in Colorado, he said, was "not at the top of my list of things I would redo."[34]

PESTICIDE USE: "A PUBLIC SAFETY ISSUE"

During prohibition—without regulations to contend with and in need of serious solutions to fight problems such as spider mites and powdery mildew that are inevitable in monoculture indoor grows—many cannabis cultivators came to rely on harsh synthetic pesticides and fungicides that were not approved for human consumption. As more states voted to legalize cannabis and companies set up massive grows, officials struggled to figure out how to deal with those ubiquitous chemicals.

In Oregon, where voters legalized adult use of cannabis in 2014, the Cannabis Safety Institute found pesticide residues exceeding allowable levels for an agricultural product on close to half of the retail products it tested in 2015. Pesticide use was increasing tremendously as growers fought diseases spread across states by a surge in sales of immature clones, CSI stated in a white paper. "Given that cannabis production has developed and operated in an unregulated setting, various practices have been adopted that are at odds with accepted regulations regarding human safety and environmental impacts," the paper stated. "Chief amongst these is the unregulated use of pesticides, which has potentially serious public health and environmental consequences." CSI found roughly ten times the level of pesticides in concentrates as in flower, indicating that extraction techniques distill pesticides as well as terpenes and cannabinoids.[35]

SC Labs, a company that tested cannabis in Oregon and California, found the presence of pesticides that were not approved for use on cannabis in three to four of every ten samples it tested.[36] Though California was the first state to legalize medical marijuana in 1996, it didn't start requiring testing for pesticides and contaminants until a year after adult-use sales began in 2018. In 2017, when Steep Hill Labs tested forty-four samples from Los Angeles dispensaries, it found that forty-one—93 percent—tested positive for pesticides at levels that would have caused them to be banned in states that regulated pesticides in cannabis products. "It appears pesticides are very widely used," said Dr. Don Land, Steep Hill's chief scientist. "It was surprising that so many [samples] had so much contamination."[37]

Lewis Koski, deputy director of enforcement for the Colorado Department of Revenue, which oversees Colorado's cannabis industry, said regulating pesticide use was "a very challenging area of policy," but added, "It's really important because it really is a public safety issue."[38]

Colorado governor John Hickenlooper was well aware. In 2015, he issued an executive order declaring that cannabis grown using unauthorized pesticides was a threat to public safety and must be removed from commerce and destroyed. The Denver Department of Public Health created a cannabis sustainability work group to look at the issue, and Denver health officials issued more than twenty recalls of cannabis products for pesticide contamination, mostly based on traces of Dow Chemical's Eagle 20, which releases hydrogen cyanide—a poisonous gas—when heated. The failure rate for cannabis samples tested for unapproved pesticides fell dramatically.

Colorado couldn't turn to the federal government for help, because as long as cannabis remained federally illegal, the US Food and Drug Administration could not enforce organic standards as it did for the food industry. In the absence of federal oversight, a few organizations stepped in to offer third-party certification for growers using organic cultivation methods. The nonprofit Cannabis Certification Council offered a national certification program and seal for organic cultivation and fair labor practices in both the United States and Canada; California-based Clean Green Certified offered certifications that mimicked federal organic standards in California, Washington, Oregon, Nevada, and Colorado; and Certified Kind followed standards equivalent to the internationally accepted norms for organic crops and processed products in Oregon, Nevada, California, Colorado, and Washington.

CANNABIS DINING: FROM PIZZA AND CHEESECAKE TO WILD BOAR STEW AND CHOCOLATE BUTTER

When the first wave of entrepreneurs rushed into business in Colorado after the Cole Memo was issued in 2009, Steve Horwitz was right there. That year, he opened Ganja Gourmet, a restaurant serving a full menu of cannabis-infused food on South Broadway in Denver, to much national acclaim. (*Tonight Show* host Jay Leno joked, "I mean, you're going to order the pizza anyway . . .") Ganja Gourmet served all Horwitz's favorites: LaGanja (lasagna), Panama Red Pizza, Ganjanade (olive tapenade), infused cheesecake, and other sweets. Diners had to show their state-issued medical marijuana cards to get in, and servers wore tie-dyed T-shirts with the slogan, "Our food is so great, you need a license to eat it!!!"

It was also expensive, at $89 for a pizza and $120 for a dozen almond horns, largely because Horwitz's chef insisted on making crockpot butter extractions from cannabis flower in house rather than relying on cheaper butane or CO_2 extractions. And within a year, once the Denver City Council banned consumption of cannabis where it was sold, it was no longer legal. America's first cannabis restaurant would follow the bumpy path of legalization in Colorado, becoming a takeout place in 2010, a medical dispensary in 2011, and a medical/recreational store in 2015. "Ever since I opened this business, I've had a black cloud around me," Horwitz said. "Pretty much nothing has worked the way it should have or could have."[39]

Horwitz was hardly alone in his thwarted dreams of a cannabis restaurant. Nine years later, no one in any legal state had managed to find a way through the tangle of varying state laws, semilaws, and regulations about social cannabis consumption and cannabis-infused food to pull it off. Instead, cannabis-curious chefs across the country began putting their efforts into creating lines of branded edibles and orchestrating semisecret pop-up dinners featuring cannabis-infused cuisine.

Celebrated pastry chef and cookbook author Mindy Segal, owner of Chicago's popular Mindy's HotChocolate Restaurant and Dessert Bar, launched Mindy's First Batch, a line of culinary-quality gourmet chocolates and brittles infused with cannabis distillate (oil extracted via fractional distillation), for the Illinois medical marijuana market in 2016 (see photo on next page). Segal was the first big-name chef to put her name behind an edibles brand, and she said she did so because the feel-good food was a natural extension of why she became a chef in the first place: to make people feel happy.

Mindy's First Batch garnered plenty of adoring international attention, though the pot jokes were inevitable. "The thought of being able to purchase edibles crafted by a James Beard Award–winning chef—Segal would be the pioneer—seemed more like a stoner's dream come true than a legitimate business venture," Lauren Viera quipped in the *New York Times* when the line launched. Segal was undeterred. "I'm not the first chef to move into this space," she said, "and I won't be the last, because food and cannabis go hand in hand."[40]

Hipster favorite Roberta's in Bushwick, Brooklyn, was among the first and most famous restaurants to offer special dinners with "weed-heavy" tasting menus that included items such as Sour Diesel Kief-Seasoned Bluefish with Cannabis Yoghurt and Pumpernickel-Cannabis Croutons and Cannabis Oil Parsley Cake with Hemp Crumble. *GQ* writer Jess Pearson, a vocal critic of the unimaginative edibles available

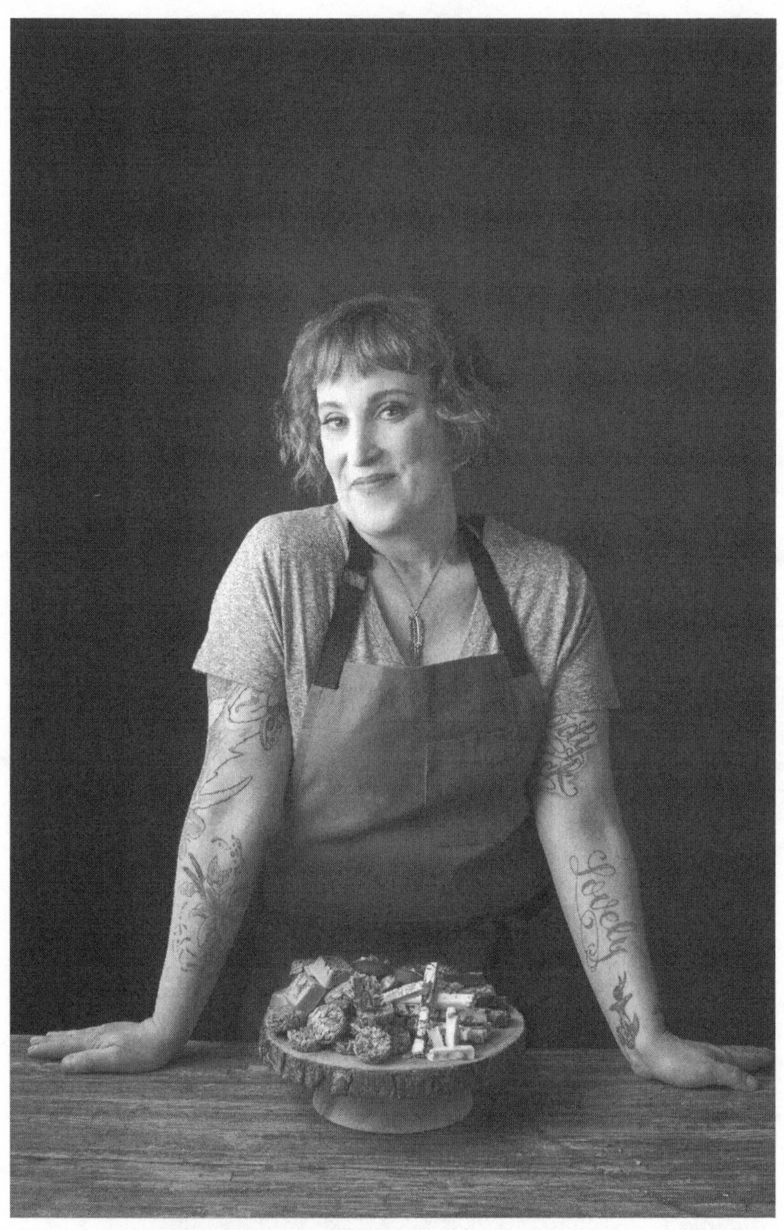

Award-winning Chicago-based chef Mindy Segal with her Mindy's Artisanal Edibles collection. Photo by Jennifer Olson Photography/Courtesy of Cresco Labs.

on dispensary shelves at that time, attended one of the dinners and was moved to declare, "I saw weed claimed in the name of great food. I saw, hopefully, the beginning of the end for the pot brownie."[41]

Jonathan Gold, the Pulitzer Prize–winning *Los Angeles Times* food critic, wrote about attending multicourse cannabis-infused dinners (like the one where McDonough sat next to him) and attributed their rise in the L.A. foodie scene to the current obsession with single, exotic ingredients. As accounts of underground supper clubs and not-so-secret pop-up dinners began to appear in mainstream media outlets from the *Los Angeles Times* to the *New Yorker*, celebrity chefs from Cat Cora to Mario Batali—whose pot brownie recipe was widely ridiculed for technical and culinary deficiencies—dipped into the possibilities of the emerging industry.

Cannabis food evolved, rapidly, from pizza and cookies to mocktails and mahi-mahi, as a rising cannabis foodie culture came to expect an elevated level of sophistication. Chefs delivered with innovations in technique and taste that no other realm of the culinary arts could match as the focus shifted from delivering the maximum amount of THC to creating balanced, nuanced, life-giving food. "It's not the goal anymore, to get you as stoned as possible by packing maximum cannabis oil into one cookie," Abdullah Saeed, who hosted the Viceland TV series *Bong Appétit*, explained. "It's an ingredient that's valuable beyond its psychoactive properties. The ultimate goal isn't just to get high; it's about a holistic eating experience."[42]

Cannabis food became a focal point for a range of culinary happenings, from farm-to-table dinners held on rooftops, in warehouses, and in open fields to elaborate productions such as the White Rabbit High Tea series in Los Angeles, where guests wearing flamboyant costumes and masks enjoyed tea and infused baked goods made by celebrity chefs and played croquet. "I want our guests to walk into something they have never experienced before and walk away talking about it for months," White Rabbit founder Jessica Cole told cannabis lifestyle website *Merry Jane*. "It's always so intriguing to see who will come to each tea event—from celebrities and tastemakers/influencers to cannabis industry professionals to moms trying cannabis for the first time."[43]

Los Angeles–based Chris Sayegh, who trained at Michelin restaurants before he became a public ambassador for cannabis cuisine (and a media darling) as The Herbal Chef, grew his business from a private dinner booked by an Instagram follower to a catering business producing $350 a plate, ten-course dinners around the world. Sayegh's dinners featured French fare with Italian and Middle Eastern influences, including Lamb Chops with THC-Infused Mint Chutney, Hamachi, and Caviar; Asparagus with Hemp Seed; Broccoli with THC-Infused Habanero Mousse and Dandelion Puree; and his signature Lamb Wellington with Spice Rub, Mint Pesto, and THC-Infused Lamb Jus.[44] A proponent of foraging, fishing, and hunting for ingredients in order to connect diners with the land around them, Sayegh's goal was to showcase local farmers and producers wherever he was cooking for people.

Like a shaman performing ritual healing, Sayegh conducted every dinner, explaining at the beginning how the night would go and how diners could expect to feel as they consumed the meal he'd engineered to keep them in what he called the "euphoric zone." Sometimes he introduced mood-enhancing centerpieces, swirling bowls of terpene vapors that were chosen specifically to stimulate the diners' minds and appetites. After dinner, guests retreated to a decompression lounge, where they could wipe their faces with cold eucalyptus-scented towels, get a massage, and enjoy CBD-infused petits fours to balance out the meal's THC.

Sayegh dreamed of bringing this concept to a permanent location, and he began drawing up plans for Herb, a restaurant where he could serve seasonal cannabis-infused food in a relaxing environment with art, plants, and natural lighting, as early as 2010. It took him at least eight years to get it open (it hadn't opened as of May 2018), a process that entailed lobbying first for adult use and then for social consumption legislation as well as legal battles with local officials. Sayegh and The Herbal Chef team had a direct role in writing the language for on-site consumption laws in West Hollywood and was doing the same for Canada.

It would be the world's first cannabis restaurant, if you don't count Ganja Gourmet, and Sayegh was aware of the responsibility that came with "creating a new type of immersive dining experience, paving the way for what one day will become commonplace in the culinary and cannabis scene."[45] He told *Forbes*, "We are a role model; we are setting the standard for how all cannabis restaurants are gonna function after us, to make sure they're safe, make sure that people are properly dosed, people are taken care of. . . . Herb is gonna be the culmination of everything we've learned, all the data that we've gathered over the years."[46]

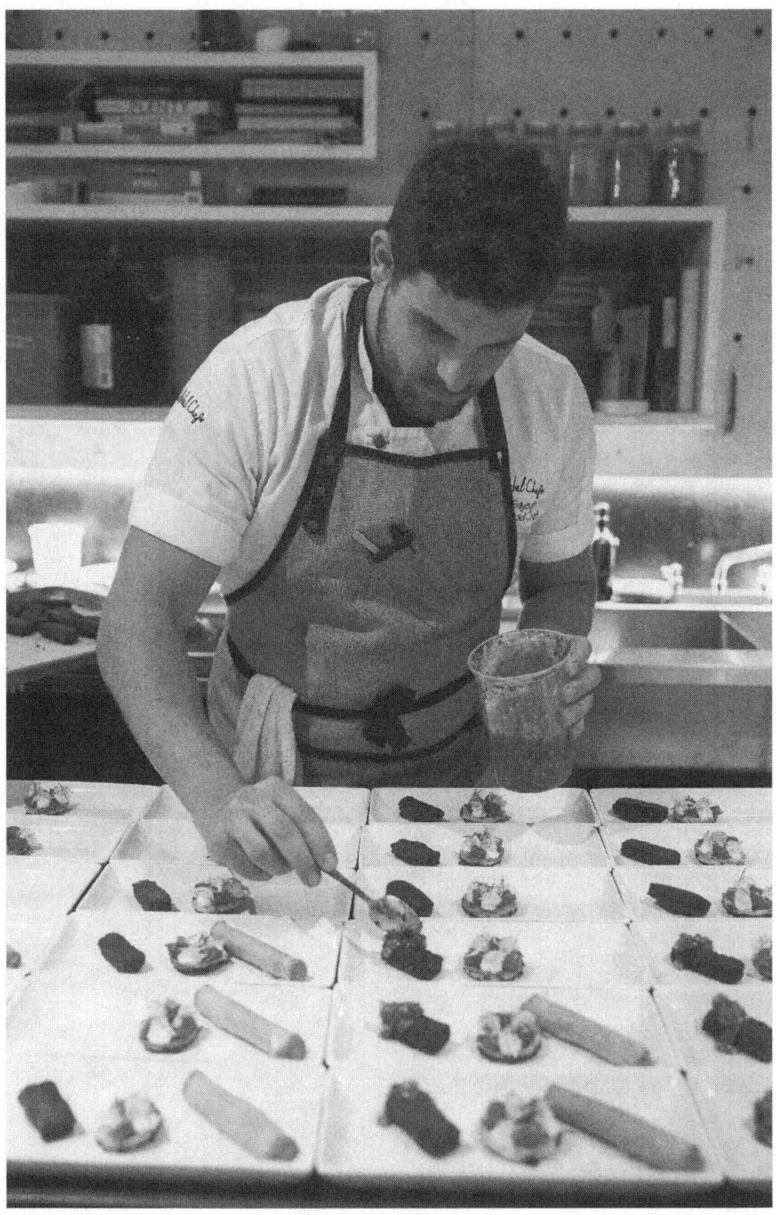

Chris Sayegh, who calls himself The Herbal Chef, caters upscale cannabis dinners around the world.

In the meantime, there were pop-up dinners. The number of semisecret pop-up dinners featuring well-known chefs and artfully made cannabis-infused food and drinks—of as fine a quality as you would find in any five-star restaurant—exploded in the 2010s. For $150 per plate in San Francisco, The Cannaisseur Series offered dishes such as cannabis-infused Spinach Arancini with Smoked Mozzarella, Wild Boar Sausage Stew, and Bread Pudding with Cardamom Caramel Sauce and Gorilla Glue Hydrosol Bourbon Vanilla Cream,[47] and Michael Magallanes's Opulent Chef offered cannabis-infused French Toast Sticks with Sea Urchin and Pickled Rhubarb and Coffee-Roasted Carrots with Savory Chocolate Ganache infused with Hash Coconut Oil and Dried Chiles.[48]

In San Diego, the Closed Door Supper Club lured in cannabis gourmets with seasonal pop-up dinners in secret locations featuring dishes such as Tempura Cannabis Leaves with Salted Honey; Pumpkin Pie Shooters with CBD-Infused Peppermint Foam; Pork Belly Cooked in THC Butter; and Pecan Cupcakes with CBD-Infused Chocolate Whiskey Syrup.[49] "Cannabis dinners have been happening for years," said Marie Daniels, the club's founder, in 2017. "I simply wanted to

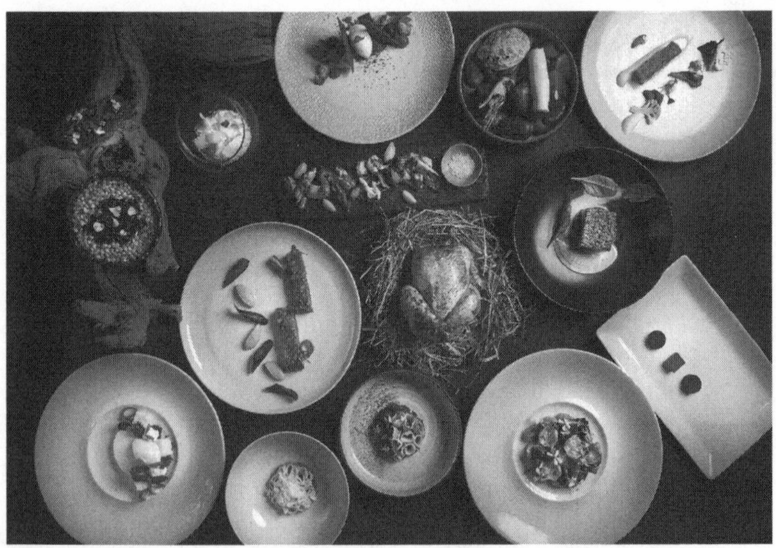

A cannabis-infused meal prepared by Chris Sayegh, The Herbal Chef.

peel away the Cheech and Chong stigma and combine the element of fine dining into the cannabis experience in an approachable way."[50]

In Chicago, where a strict and poorly supported medical marijuana program made for an anemic cannabis cuisine scene, diners lined up for $125 tickets to pop-up dinners sponsored by San Diego–based Herbal Notes, which featured dishes such as Crispy Pig-Head Croquette with Black-Bean Puree and Watermelon Haze Thyme Salt; Tamal with Cranberry-Ginger Reduction, Roasted Sweet Potato, and Cherry Kandahar Pepper; and Swordfish Ceviche with Watermelon Haze Keef-Tajin Seasoning.[51] In Philadelphia, where medical marijuana was legalized in 2016 but dispensaries didn't open until two years later, beloved local chef David Ansill emerged to fill a market void with infused versions of the decadent dishes he was known for throughout the city, such as Salmon Tartare with Cannabis-Infused Chile Oil; Crostini Smeared with Bone Marrow Whipped with Ganja Butter; Grilled Marinated Quail with "Medicated" Jamaican Rum; and *Marquise de Chocolat* Drizzled with Cannabis-Infused *Mirabelle eau de Vie*, which the chef described as "basically chocolate butter."[52]

New Yorkers, famous around the world for their love of gastronomical explorations, couldn't get enough of the dinners and brunches created by a robust circuit of locally renowned chefs and entrepreneurial pioneers. Because cannabis use for adults was still illegal there, the secret locations of the speakeasy-style pop-up dinners were often not revealed until days or even hours before the events. Miguel Trinidad, whose modern Filipino restaurant Maharlika was the talk of the town less than a year after it launched as a (noncannabis) pop-up in 2011, led the way with 99th Floor, which offered semimonthly invitation-only dinners featuring cannabis-infused fusion dishes such as *Vitello Tonnato* (cold veal loin brushed with cannabis-infused coconut oil); Smoked *Bangus* (milkfish) Mousse with Capers Fried in Cannabis Coconut Oil; and Slow-Cooked Pork Belly Braised in Cannabis-Infused Oil and Butter with Star Anise, Fermented Black Bean, and Tamari.[53]

New Yorkers "Hawaii" Mike and Stephanie Salman, who were not chefs, smelled opportunity and then tasted it, producing monthly cannabis dinners in secret locations through their company Chef for Higher, which attracted diverse crowds of teachers, DJs, foodies, creative professionals, and attorneys. The Salmans' goal, in addition to making money, was to create awareness and community around can-

Celebrity Edibles

When cannabis edibles opened up as a whole new, very lucrative market opportunity in the 2010s, America's A-listers were right up front to get their share. Not surprisingly, renowned stoners Snoop Dogg and Willie Nelson were two of the first to bite, with stoner icon Whoopi Goldberg not far behind.

Snoop Dogg's cannabis company, Leafs by Snoop, offered a line of hard candies, gummies, fruit chews, peanut butter gems, and confectionary bars alongside the brand's signature wax, shatter, and flower, and Nelson's company, Willie's Reserve, soon followed with chocolates and hard candies branded by Nelson's wife, Annie, to round out its flower and vaping offerings.

Goldberg teamed up with award-winning edibles maker Maya Elisabeth to create a signature line of herbal medical cannabis products formulated to provide relief for menstrual cramps and muscle aches, including a cannabis-infused raw cacao and agave morsel.

nabis, they said. "At the end of alcohol prohibition in New York, there were more than 2,200 speakeasies, and that's where we got the idea. We thought, it's New York, you know how much stuff happens behind closed doors?" Mike Salman said. "We wanted to recreate that because it's the same place we're at right now with cannabis prohibition."[54]

Some chefs and restaurateurs didn't want to wait for cannabis to be fully legalized and laws regarding social consumption to change, so they found a workaround, taking baby steps by infusing food with hemp, cannabis strains that skirted under the law because they delivered large amounts of the nonpsychoactive cannabinoid CBD and very little psychoactive THC.

Arizona-based chef Payton Curry held a pop-up event called Cannavore featuring CBD-infused *maitake* steaks and sweet corn tamales topped with medicated *mole negro* in San Francisco before adult use was legalized in California, and a pop-up dinner at Lalito in New York's Chinatown featured CBD-infused chayote squash panzanella and Brie flan. In Portland, Oregon, Coalition Brewing had CBD-infused beers on tap, and San Diego's Madison on Park offered the Mr. Nice Guy, an $18 cocktail maid from mescal, CBD oil, matcha, pineapple, coconut milk, and lime.

Hemp was also the star at Denmark's Dragsholm Castle, where head chef Claus Henriksen used it liberally in dishes such as Sausages Stuffed with Dried Hemp Leaves and Chopped Hazelnuts and Hemp-Smoked Soft Cheese Stuffed with Fresh Hemp Leaves, served with Roasted Hemp Seed Puree. "I actually believe hemp has the ability to accentuate a lot of food," said Henriksen, who likened the taste to pistachio nuts. "You can sauté it like spinach, fry it, or cook it like creamed kale."[55]

SPAIN: "WE BUILD LITTLE FANTASIES TO DANCE ARTFULLY AROUND THEM"

Because of its location just nine miles across the Strait of Gibraltar from Morocco, Spain has been a port of entry for Moroccan hashish into Western Europe for centuries. Spain was tolerant of cannabis for much of its modern history, until—as with so many other countries—it was pressured into joining the 1961 UN Single Convention on Narcotics.

Spain outlawed cannabis in 1967, then followed up in 1973 by changing the penal code to make drug possession of any kind a punishable offense. This move triggered a lawsuit that went to the Supreme Court, which ruled that cases of cannabis possession for self-consumption could not be prosecuted. Nine years later, the government decriminalized all drug use and established a two-tiered system for enforcing laws against "hard" drugs such as heroin, cocaine, and LSD, and "soft" drugs such as cannabis, methaqualone, flunitrazepam, and alprazolam.

Selling cannabis for profit continued to be a serious offense, but that didn't stop Moroccan hashish from continuing to flood the Spanish market. The government again cracked down in 1992 with a decree that anyone carrying cannabis in public could be searched and fined. Even though cannabis was, officially, decriminalized, 300,000 people were fined for using drugs, mostly cannabis, between 1997 and 2002. Tens of thousands of Spaniards who wished to consume cannabis but didn't want to expose themselves to potential police harassment and street dealers turned in droves to home cultivation.

In 1998, according to a *High Times* report by author and grower Jorge Cervantes (George Van Patten), the legendary Australian breeder Scott Blakey, aka Shantibaba, sprinkled Spain with twenty-five thousand seeds of White Widow, White Shark, California Orange, and Haze crosses—strains he had created for the seed company he cofounded and left in The Netherlands—forever changing the gene pool.[56] By the early 2000s, secret cannabis plantations were flourishing under the abundant sunlight on once-fallow farms all along Spain's Mediterranean coast,[57] and by 2013 this domestic crop had replaced Moroccan imports as the country's primary source of cannabis.

As in many other European countries, Spain was home to an active cannabis rights movement that grew up in the 1990s, and a few of them took advantage of provisions in Spanish law that allowed for private cultivation and shared consumption as the basis for founding the country's first cannabis club, *Club de Catadores de Cannabis de Barcelona*, a noncommercial collective that pooled its resources to grow cannabis for members' personal consumption in members-only establishments, in 2001. Club de Catadores was immediately slapped with lawsuits, which led to several Supreme Court rulings in its favor, paving the way for cannabis enthusiasts in cities throughout Spain to start their own clubs.

By the early 2000s, Spain was becoming known around the world for its cannabis clubs, ranging in style from hippie living rooms to sleek wellness centers to a famous Barcelona collective open only to women in their eighties, all of them offering cannabis, hashish, and sometimes a paltry selection of space cakes for members' shared consumption on the premises. The clubs registered as legal entities and followed self-imposed regulations stating that members must be eighteen or older and not first-time users. Members were supposed to provide a local residential address, though tourists found this easy to get around, and pay a small yearly fee for their share of the harvest.

Though the clubs didn't advertise in traditional outlets, memberships could be found and procured over the Internet. Travel writer Rick Steves reported that this was a type of system familiar to Spaniards, who often told him, "We are used to dealing with old laws that should be changed but don't. We build little fantasies to dance artfully around them."[58]

Spain's different provinces were allowed to set strict rules for the clubs or ban them altogether, and many municipalities did. Most were clustered in Catalonia, where rules were most lenient, and the clubs often reflected their regions. "In the northern Basque region, they're informal meeting places where the famous cured hams are shared with bread and wine. In Madrid and Barcelona, they can be quite fancy, with multiple levels of clean, well-appointed rooms, including framed artworks," Danny Danko reported in *High Times*.[59] By 2014, Catalonia was home to more than five hundred cannabis social clubs (three hundred in Barcelona alone) with more than 165,00 members[60] and an industry association with a code of conduct based on "transparency, democracy, and non-profitability."[61]

Barcelona became known as "the Amsterdam of southern Europe" and, as The Netherlands began taking measures to discourage tourist traffic at its famed coffee houses, "the new Amsterdam." Spannabis and the World Cannabis Conferences, held the second weekend of every March starting in 2004, brought more than thirty thousand cannabis enthusiasts and five hundred vendors to Barcelona for an expo that rivaled Northern California's famed Emerald Cup as the world's largest.[62] By 2015, some seventy-five cannabis social clubs had opened up in London and another four hundred in France.[63]

In 2017, the year consumers were estimated to have spent about one billion euros in Spain's more than seven hundred cannabis clubs,[64] the Catalonian government voted overwhelmingly to regulate cannabis clubs, making provisions to oversee transportation, packaging, hygienic storage, testing, and distribution of the cannabis that clubs cultivated for members. As the cannabis social club industry took another step toward legitimacy, a few companies saw what was happening in other legal markets and began selling cannabis-infused lollipops and drinks. The edibles industry in Spain was born.

URUGUAY: "SOMEONE HAS TO BE THE FIRST"

Another country that had always been tolerant of cannabis, Uruguay did what was required to comply after it was coerced into joining the 1961 UN Single Convention on Narcotic Drugs, while at the same time taking a hands-off approach in practice. In 1974, the country decriminalized drug possession for personal use, but cannabis arrests still occurred with plenty of frequency.

In 2011, Alicia Castilla, a sixty-six-year-old who was growing cannabis in her home, was arrested, triggering a huge public outcry. Uruguay's Brownie Mary brought cannabis legalization to the nation's

Spain's Brownie Mary

Fernanda de la Figuera, often referred to as Spain's "grandmother of marijuana activism," was the first person to test Spanish laws permitting cultivation for personal use in 1995 after the farm in Andalusia where she grew cannabis and made her own tinctures, concentrates, and edibles was raided.

De la Figuera's victory in the courts made her the country's first legal cannabis farmer. She founded *Marias Para Maria* (Mothers for Marijuana), a cannabis club committed to giving women safe, easy access to cannabis as well as offering informal cultivation training, talks about cannabis legislation, and a place to commune.

"I think people really listen to senior women because we've been working with this stuff for years," de la Figuera said. "We just know about marijuana, and if there were problems with it, we'd know about them as well."

Source: Caitlin Donohue, "La Abuela: Fernanda de la Figuera Is Spain's Grandmother of Marijuana," *SF Evergreen*, May 20, 2015, http://sfevergreen.com/la-abuela-fernanda-de-la-figuera-is-spains-grandmother-of-marijuana/.

attention. A deep grassroots movement made up mostly of middle-class cannabis consumers came together to march and protest at open-air reggae concerts, and they caught the attention of President José Mujica, who was called the world's poorest president, a former guerrilla who gained international attention for living in a humble shack, giving most of his salary to charity, and wearing sandals. Though he said he never used cannabis himself, Mujica understood the problems prohibition had caused.

Mujica presented a bill to legalize adult use of cannabis to congress in late 2012, saying legalization was the only answer to the drug-related violence that was shattering much of Latin America. "I'm scared by the drug trafficking, not by the drug," Mujica told the BBC.[65] Other Latin American states, including Colombia, Guatemala, and Mexico, were enacting or considering measures to legalize medical marijuana and decriminalize adult use, but no country in the world had taken a step so bold. "Someone has to be the first," Mujica told the *Guardian*.[66]

Mujica pushed through his bill, which called for state-run cannabis production, despite tepid public support for cannabis legalization. When it passed in 2013, the bill had been altered considerably. Instead of growing its own, the government licensed private growers to produce price-regulated cannabis that could be sold only in pharmacies to Uruguayan citizens who were registered users. These users could purchase up to forty grams per month from pharmacies, register to grow up to six plants of their own, or join cooperatives to grow collectively. The bill created the world's first state-run cannabis marketplace, and it wasn't easy to implement or without controversy.

Many cannabis users found the new law's extreme regulations, arbitrary limits on consumption, and paper trails draconian. Many saw the registration requirement as an invasion of privacy. Polls consistently found that most Uruguayans—60 to 66 percent—opposed cannabis regulation. They were more in favor of legalizing medical marijuana, which Mujica criticized for potentially "brutal hypocrisy."[67] Julio Calzada, a public health official who helped write Uruguay's regulations, spoke for many when he said he was afraid the nation would become like Colorado, a "competitive industry peddling pot versions of Marlboro and Camel."[68]

Nevertheless, on the day the law took effect in July 2017, registered users lined up at the sixteen pharmacies across Uruguay that offered cannabis and came out proudly displaying blue and white envelopes with labels verifying the authenticity and warning about the effects of the fragrant green flowers inside. They paid $1.30 per gram. Two government-sanctioned growers received ninety cents of that, and the rest was split between the pharmacies and government drug-prevention programs.

Later that year, the government began registering cannabis growers' clubs, allowing up to forty-five members to cultivate up to ninety-nine plants and personally receive up to forty grams (1.4 ounces) every month. The collectives put up huge greenhouses around the capital of Montevideo where members could tend to their plants and test the harvest, giving smokers a social outlet—a highly regulated version of Spain's cannabis social clubs.[69]

The government's apparent goal, wrote *Washington Post* reporter Nick Miroff, was "to make marijuana use as boring as possible." There were no Amsterdam-style cafés or "shops selling ganja candies, psychedelic pastries, or any of the other derivatives."[70] There were only restaurants like Montevideo's Hemp-T Café, where advertisements promised that diners could learn about "the new and exciting world of cannabis," but it was not on the menu.

Uruguay's program had problems. Price controls left pharmacists with barely any profit and therefore little incentive to carry state-sanctioned cannabis, leaving many Uruguayans with no choice but the black market—which was also buoyed by tourists, who were locked out of the legal market. Uruguayan police seized almost three times as much black-market cannabis in 2017 as they had before legalization, while neighbors Brazil and Argentina reported seizing more Uruguayan homegrown.[71]

Uruguay, where hemp plantations dated to the eighteenth century when the country was still under colonial rule, was also eager to get its piece of the billion-dollar global hemp market. Four companies were given permits to produce hemp, and a fledgling industry of CBD-infused edibles, offering everything from the traditional sweets to *yerba mate*, emerged as tiny Uruguay sought to take the lead in a legal cannabis market expected to be worth $776 million in South America by 2027.

• 6 •

Future Feast or Famine?

When Proposition 215 legalizing medical marijuana passed in California, the voter initiative attempted to stifle commercialization of the market by stipulating that cannabis businesses could not turn a profit and limiting the number of plants farmers could grow as well as the number of small farm licenses an entity could have—two hindrances that went a long way toward preventing the state's "green rush" from getting any larger than it did.

California—the world's fifth largest economy—was already the world's largest legal cannabis market when the California Department of Food and Agriculture eliminated those rules in 2016, opening up the state's cannabis industry to corporate interests and out-of-state investors and terrifying the small farmers and grassroots businesspeople who had ruled the industry for twenty years. "Marlboro can go put up a thousand-fucking-acre grow if they want to," Chris Anderson, whose family had grown cannabis in Humboldt County for generations, told Zach Sokol in *Playboy*.[1]

The race was on, as investors sought out growers, manufacturers, and retailers who could pump out the massive amounts of cannabis and cannabis products the state's thriving medical marijuana market had already proven it could absorb. The price of land tripled in tumbleweed-choked towns such as Adelanto and Desert Hot Springs, which were quick to approve large-scale grows in hopes of refilling empty coffers. "People are definitely salivating over the California market," Troy Dayton, chief executive of research and investment services firm Arcview Group, told the *New York Times* in April 2016. "It's huge, and Californians love cannabis so much."[2]

Not everyone was as thrilled. In a *Los Angeles Times* article about California being poised to become the center of cannabis culture a month later, former *High Times* editor and *Bong Appétit* producer David Bienenstock, a former *High Times* editor, lamented, "Prohibition, for all its evils, acted in a way to protect this underground economy from capitalism."[3]

Then, in November 2016, the big event happened. Fifty-seven percent of California voters approved Proposition 64, legalizing adult use of cannabis. Analysts and industry pundits went wild. *The New Yorker* predicted California's influence would kick cannabis into the realm of "the booming wellness industry."[4]

New Frontier Data predicted adult-use sales alone would be $1.1 billion in their first year, and would rise to $3.1 billion, usurping medical marijuana sales of $2.5 billion by 2020.[5] *Business Insider*'s headline promised California's cannabis market would "soar to $5.1 billion—and it's going to be bigger than beer." Based on research from BDS Analytics, the article predicted sales would reach $3.7 billion by the end of 2018 and more than $5.1 billon by 2019.[6] Industry pundits promised the cash-strapped state a $185 million tax windfall in the first six months alone.[7]

In 2016, according to Arcview Group, edible sales in California were about $180 million—a number everyone expected to grow exponentially once the state put the regulatory framework for adult use in place, allowing the market to mature.[8] Until adult use was implemented, California edibles manufacturers had been given more or less free reign, with no regulations on THC content, testing, labeling, or packaging. When the newly established Bureau of Medical Cannabis Regulation released a set of proposed regulations for that framework in 2017, they were no joke.

Cannabis edibles could not contain more than ten milligrams of THC per serving, and single products could not contain more than one hundred milligrams of THC. Edibles that contained alcohol, caffeine, or had to be refrigerated or microwaved were forbidden. Child-proof packaging had to include the words *cannabis-infused*, a big red THC! triangle label, and other safety warnings. "By 2019," *LAist* reported, "the freewheeling California cannabis bonanza will be over, forever."[9]

For twenty years, all it had taken was access to cannabis and a few good recipes to launch an edibles business, and plenty of people had.

The new rules, however, meant the end of the cottage industry of mom-and-pop brownie bakers and craft confection makers that had grown up in California's lawless yet quasi-legal medical marijuana market. When that gray market was forced to go completely legit in 2017, only twenty-eight edibles companies—surely a fraction of the companies responsible for $1.8 million in sales—had even the most basic state license to infuse food with cannabis.[10]

Many of the smaller edibles companies didn't have the means to move to professional kitchens—where in some municipalities rent could be nearly triple the going rate as city zoning officials clustered cannabis businesses into real estate–scarce "green zones"—or to change packaging and dosing to become compliant with the new regulations. For companies that had made their names on the astronomical potency of their products—some candy bars packed a whopping one thousand milligrams of THC—the regulations were a disaster. Harborside CEO Steve DeAngelo called the new rules an "extinction event" and predicted they would knock 75 percent of existing edibles companies out of business.[11]

By January 2018, just as the state officially opened up adult-use sales, Elise McDonough reported on *Vice* that hundreds of small edibles manufacturers were "closing up shop or returning to the underground." Among the victims was Auntie Delores, a beloved line of nuts, crackers, and vegan sweets that couldn't be easily divided into ten-milligram serving sizes. Auntie Delores founder Julianna Carella complained that the only way to comply with the regulations was to make chocolates or candies, which she emphatically would not make.

Matthew Gill of cannabis-infused artisanal cheese company THCheese was crushed when he found out his product was no longer viable under the no-dairy rule, he told McDonough. "We made farm-to-table edibles with a focus on fermentation, showcasing the agricultural side of food and cannabis. These types of products were viewed as dangerous due to their perishability and the risk of food-borne pathogens."[12] Singer-songwriter Melissa Etheridge, who had introduced a line of cannabis-infused wine in 2014, was the only company in the state to dodge the no-alcohol rule when she renamed her product Know Label Wine Tincture and sold it only to medical marijuana patients.[13]

The opening of the world's largest legal cannabis marketplace on January 1, 2018, grabbed the world's attention, and long lines formed to access newly opened adult-use stores across the state—but the rollout was far from flawless. Political and bureaucratic delays meant that only four stores were licensed for adult use in Los Angeles on the day adult sales began, and dozens continued to operate without a license as they had before. (State officials sent cease and desist letters to the dispensaries as well as Weedmaps, the website and app that helped patients and consumers find them.)

Six out of seven cities banned adult-use cannabis stores, and only one out of three municipalities decided cannabis businesses were welcome.[14] The industry blossomed in Oakland and San Diego, while Bakersfield and Orange County became legal cannabis desserts.

Again, people lined up around the block to be among the first adults to buy cannabis from legal stores, and the media convened on the state to document the opening of the world's largest legal cannabis market—and sales were surprisingly sluggish. Sticker-shocked consumers posted receipts showing astronomical sales and state taxes—in addition to the state's 15 percent levy on purchases of cannabis and cannabis products, local taxes and fees could add up to a tax bill of 28 to 40 percent[15]—on social media, and a slew of news articles followed. During the first two months of recreational sales, amid reports of a still-thriving black market in California, legal cannabis sales were $339 million—13 percent behind the $383 million BDS Analytics had set as the bar.[16]

Assemblyman Evan Low, who chaired the California State Assembly's Business and Professions Committee, complained that the numbers were "abysmally below" what Californians were promised when they voted to legalize recreational cannabis and warned, "The state must take all possible action to defeat the black market and support good actors, or else our newly established regulatory scheme will surely fail."[17]

CANADA: "I DON'T THINK WE'LL SEE GUMMY BEARS. EVER."

In 2015, Justin Trudeau, the telegenic young leader of Canada's Liberal Party, was elected prime minister based on a progressive platform that included legalizing cannabis—a promise he methodically began to fulfill as soon as he took office, putting the country on track to become the first G7 nation to free the plant. In 2017, flanked by Canada's ministers of health, justice, public safety, and national revenue and a former police chief, Trudeau announced the Cannabis Act, set to take effect on July 1, 2018, that would legalize access to cannabis for adults in Canada and control and regulate how it was grown, distributed, and sold. Prohibition, Trudeau said, "does not protect our young people, and it sends billions per year to organized crime and street gangs."[18]

Investors went wild as the media liberally tossed around Deloitte's estimate that the market for legal cannabis in Canada would be worth at least $5 billion in 2018, with ancillary goods and services racking up another $20 billion.[19] (To put that in perspective, Canadians spent the same amount on spirits and $7 billion on wine in 2017.[20]) "Canada is the tenth largest economy in the world, and the first major economy to legalize cannabis," said Troy Dayton, CEO of investor service and market research firm Arcview. "There's no state-federal conflict as there is in the U.S. We're very excited about it, and so is the Canadian government."[21]

Historically, it was quite the turnaround. Though Canadians had grown quite tolerant of cannabis use by the 2000s, particularly in British Columbia, Canada was a high-profile leader in international antinarcotic and prohibition efforts in the early twentieth century, and its criminal laws—triggered largely by anti-immigrant racism designed to keep Chinese laborers out of the country—were harsh. In the 1920s, law officers could conduct searches without warrants, and convicted drug users were whipped, given mandatory minimum sentences of hard labor, and deported.[22] Though the government antinarcotics campaign was targeted at Chinese immigrants who trafficked and used opium, Parliament added cannabis to the schedule of restricted drugs under the Narcotics Control Act in 1923 after a vigorous smear campaign whipped up anticannabis sentiment.

Emily Murphy, also known as Janey Canuck, the police magistrate and juvenile court judge for Edmonton, spearheaded the propaganda with a series of articles in *MacLean's* warning that young women would give in to Chinese men's sexual demands and have mixed-race babies while under the influence of hashish. Her enormously influential 1922 book, *The Black Candle*, cites Alexandre Dumas's *The Count of Monte Cristo* and Fitz Hugh Ludlow's *The Hasheesh Eater* in illustrating the horrors of hashish and claimed this "new menace" turned users into raving maniacs who were "liable to kill or indulge in any sort of violence to other persons, using the most savage methods of cruelty without . . . any sense of moral responsibility."[23]

Canadians were horrified by this new drug, hashish, and most had no idea it had anything to do with the hemp they grew as windbreakers around their properties. Royal Canadian Mounted Police officers reported that people were shocked when they made sweeps and told them they had to eradicate the plants in the 1930s. When they told an older woman she would have to destroy the plants she grew to feed her canaries, she chased the Mounties away with a broom.[24]

In the late 1960s and 1970s, cannabis came to Canada with the hippies, and the courts and prisons became overloaded with cannabis offenders serving mandatory six-month sentences. Canada joined several other nations in relaxing cannabis laws and lifted mandatory imprisonment in 1969. Prime Minister Pierre Trudeau, Justin's father, foreshadowed his son's move in the late 1970s, saying, "If you have a joint and you're smoking it for your private pleasure, you shouldn't be hassled."

Fewer people went to jail, but cannabis continued to be the focus of Canadian law enforcement efforts throughout the 1970s and 1980s. Brian Mulroney, the Progressive Conservative prime minister who was elected after Pierre Trudeau, was one of the first to jump on the bandwagon when US president Ronald Reagan led the United States and the world into the war on drugs in 1986. Mulroney announced that drug use had become an "epidemic that undermines our economic as well as our social fabric," gave police new powers to seize drug offenders' assets, and banned the sale of all drug paraphernalia (which meant the end, even, of *High Times* magazine in Canada).[25]

In 2000, a Canadian court ruled that it was the government's duty to make medical marijuana available to citizens. It did so in 2001, unleashing a chaotic free-for-all period not unlike what happened in California and Colorado as a flood of small growers stepped in to supply patients and play the system. In 2014, the government stepped in with strict regulations requiring patients to buy cannabis only from approved for-profit producers, the first step toward consolidating the new industry and shutting down thousands of informal growing operations throughout Canada.[26]

In the original legislation, Canadian authorities had allowed only for the sale of dried cannabis flower and nothing else, and again the matter went to the Supreme Court, which ruled that patients had a right to consume medical marijuana in whatever manner they preferred. This gave licensed producers the go-ahead to start producing edible cannabis oil, though premade edibles remained illegal. About forty thousand Canadians registered as patients,[27] which wasn't always necessary. In many areas, buying cannabis was as easy as walking into a dispensary and filling out a form that included checking off a box about the patient's medical condition. Unlicensed dispensaries were as common in Canada as they were in California.

Determined not to make the same mistakes that California and Colorado had, Bill Blair, the former Toronto police chief who headed Justin Trudeau's task force on legalization, sought out and received plenty of candid advice from jurisdictions that had legalized, leading him to adopt a regulatory approach that *The Spectator* writer Danny Kruger called "as square as possible." Cannabis products would be sold in plain packages and could not appeal to children, be advertised, or sold alongside alcohol and tobacco. Taxes would be based on potency. "It is, one must admit, all rather joyless," Kruger wrote. "But after all, cannabis is joyless stuff. The Canadians are simply applying their national formula—liberal and boring at the same time—to a problem that deserves it."[28]

Though edibles were widely available in licensed and unlicensed dispensaries throughout Canada and online, in 2017 the government chose to delay the complex undertaking of designing a regulatory system for edibles until July 2019. Only cannabis flowers, oils, seeds, and plants for cultivation were approved for legal commerce. Though many predicted edibles would eventually make up the largest piece of the Canadian cannabis market, an Ottawa lawyer who specialized in cannabis told the *Toronto Sun*, "I don't think we'll see gummy bears in Canada. Ever."[29] Health Canada planned to promote healthier edible options such as cannabis-infused kombucha and protein drinks.[30]

Marijuana Policy Group cofounder Miles Light told CBC News that edibles and nonflower products were the ultimate endgame for cannabis and pointed out that cannabis food was a friendlier niche for new and smaller companies than cannabis production, which was already dominated by a handful of mega-producers.[31] And Canadians appeared to be hungry for edibles. An Ipsos survey for Global News found that 7 percent regularly used edibles in 2017, but 29 percent (51 percent of

Canadian Happy Pizza

For a couple of years, between 2014 and 2016, hungry medical marijuana patients could show their government-issued medical cards and have cannabis oil added to their pizza for about $10 extra at Mega iLL on Kingsway in Vancouver.

Inspired by Cambodian "happy" pizzerias and restaurants, the nondescript pizza joint offered "medikated and non-medikated" pizza with hemp heart crust and cinnamon treats. Mega iLL billed itself as the "Chucky Cheese for Adults," and its website promised "healthy food in a Pot Friendly environment with a positive attitude and outlook on life."

young adults between eighteen and thirty-four) planned to try them when cannabis became legal in Canada.[32]

In September 2017, a Dalhousie University study found that 46 percent of Canadians would try cannabis-infused bakery products, candy, oil, and spices, but nearly 53 percent disagreed that it was a healthy ingredient for their diets. "The benefits of eating cannabis-infused food products aren't really clear," Sylvain Charlebois, dean of the Faculty of Management and professor in Distribution and Policy at Dalhousie University, told *Food in Canada*. "Is it really recreational? Is it just for fun? That needs to be defined, because in the whole area of functional foods, the focus has been on health. If it's not healthy, then why would you eat it in the first place?"[33]

"IT WILL BECOME A FOOD INGREDIENT"

"We're at that moment in *Thelma and Louise* when they have driven the car off the cliff," Scott Greacen, a longtime resident of Humboldt, California, where illegal cannabis growing had anchored the economy since the 1970s, told the *Washington Post* in spring of 2018. "We're just waiting for the impact."[34]

"Big Tobacco 2.0" was the impact California Growers Association executive director Hezekiah Allen predicted when his organization filed a lawsuit claiming the California Department of Food and Agriculture defied the will of the voters by allowing large-scale, industrial cannabis farms.[35] Without the resources to apply for grow licenses under the state's expensive and cumbersome new regulatory system, squeezed-out small growers banded together in organizations like the CGA and Humboldt Artisanal Branding, open only to growers who used organic methods to cultivate less than three thousand square feet of plant canopy under natural light.

Investment analysts were heralding a global cannabis market they believed could be worth $75 billion by 2030.[36] Agricultural producers and suppliers were consolidating and swarming, jockeying for position in what many feared was a race to standardize the plant so it could be mono-cropped like corn, soybeans, and yellow bananas.

Scotts Miracle Gro made no secret of its ambitions within the cannabis industry when it began to buy up companies in the hydroponics space through its wholly owned subsidiary Hawthorne Gardening Co. and airing TV commercials featuring tattooed growers working with leafy plants under neon lights. Scotts CEO Jim Hagedorn called the cannabis business the "biggest thing ever" in gardening and put his son, Chris, in charge of Hawthorne. "We're squarely focused on what's made this business successful: high-value crops," Chris Hagedorn said after the company bought a stake in indoor garden manufacturer AeroGrow International, nutrient and hydroponics system company General Hydroponics, and lighting company Gavita, among others.[37]

When Chris's father told investors and analysts that Scotts saw pesticides as one of several market opportunities within hydroponics and threw in that the company was talking with the US Environmental Protection Agency about pesticide products that could be used on cannabis,[38] it sent shivers down the spines of organic advocates. Scotts, which made Miracle-Gro nitrogen-based plant food and licensed product variations such as Monsanto's Roundup, had a history of pesticide violations, including mislabeling products with carcinogens.[39] Even more terrifying to many in the industry, Hagedorn told *Forbes* he wanted to expand Scotts' genetics research to create genetically modified (GMO) cannabis.[40]

Multinational agrochemical and agricultural biotechnology behemoth Monsanto—consistently voted one of the world's most evil corporations and one of the first companies to establish offices in Uruguay after that country legalized adult use—was a perpetual cause of angst for the people who built the cannabis industry, and for small farmers everywhere. Before the US Department of Justice approved multinational pharmaceutical conglomerate Bayer's $62.5 billion acquisition of Monsanto in the largest all-cash buyout ever in 2018, a coalition of forty-five farm groups joined together to create Farm Aid to oppose the merger. "The new company would be the world's largest vegetable seed company, world's largest cottonseed company, world's largest manufacturer and seller of herbicides, and the world's largest owner of intellectual property/patents for herbicide-tolerant traits (GMOs)," the coalition stated.[41]

What that means for the cannabis industry is that Monsanto-Bayer would be poised to develop cannabis seeds resistant to blights and Monsanto's herbicide and, through Bayer's expertise, use the plants it develops to dominate cannabis-derived pharmaceuticals, *San Francisco Weekly* reported.[42] News like that had a lot of people in the cannabis industry worried that the takeover by Big Ag and Big Pharma was imminent.

In 2016, PBS's *Nova* aired an episode about US Patent No. 9095554, which was filed by an unknown group of California growers to protect "compositions and methods for the breeding, production, processing and use of specialty cannabis"—the first time a patent was issued for the cannabis plant.[43] In a *GQ* article the next year, Amanda Chicago Lewis reported that the secretive company buying the patents was Biotech Institute LLC, and it was registering utility patents—the strongest intellectual property protection available—worth hundreds of millions of dollars in the United States and internationally.

"Utility patents are big. Scary," Mowgli Holmes, chief scientific officer for Phylos Bioscience, told Lewis. "All of cannabis could be locked up. They could sue people for growing in their own backyards." Several years earlier, Holmes founded the Cannabis Genome Project to create genetic blueprints on as many strains as possible and put them into the public domain so companies couldn't market them exclusively. Still, Lewis warned, unless the rest of the cannabis industry worked together to fight the patents, Biotech could have the market cornered in a few years.[44]

In Canada, major corporations were circling. British Columbia–based Village Farms converted a large portion of its vegetable greenhouses to cannabis,[45] and Johnson & Johnson made deals with medical labs to develop medical marijuana products.[46] Meanwhile, the handful of players who already ruled the Canadian medical marijuana market consolidated even further. Alberta-based Aurora Cannabis embarked on a string of acquisitions and hostile takeovers, including a $3.2 billion buyout of medical marijuana firm MedReleaf, to create an agro-pharma-industrial giant worth $7 billion.[47]

Canada's largest licensed cannabis producer, Canopy Growth Corp., went on an acquisition spree, buying up companies in countries with legal medical marijuana markets on five continents. When Canopy announced its $29 million acquisition of Daddy Cann Lesotho in Lesotho, the first African nation to legalize cannabis in 2017, the company outlined its ambitions in the high-altitude mountainous kingdom that boasted more than three hundred days of sunshine a year, and it sounded hauntingly colonialist. "It has ideal humidity and growing conditions for greenhouse cultivation. Together with very low operating and resource costs, this places Canopy Growth in a position to produce large quantities of high-quality medical cannabis at a low cost," the company said in a statement.[48]

In 2018, Canopy moved from the Toronto Stock Exchange to the New York Stock Exchange after its shares rose 300 percent in a year, boasting a market value of $4.7 billion. "One of the primary drivers of this listing is, as we are expanding globally, having U.S. institutional investors helps," said Canopy Growth CEO Bruce Linton. "I think the investment community has to drop the pot jokes and talk about the investment-grade opportunity."[49]

Fortune 500 food manufacturers were certainly not laughing. Many of them were eyeing edibles companies to invest in or acquire in Canada, where they could sell THC-infused products throughout the country starting in 2019. Sylvain Charlebois, dean of the Faculty of Management and professor of agri-food distribution and policy at Dalhousie University, predicted that 5 to 7 percent of all food sold in Canada, including ready-to-eat, biscuits, desserts, and other items, could contain cannabis. "You can see it as far-fetched," he said, "but within ten years, our society will have a different relationship with cannabis. It will become a food ingredient."[50]

Faith Popcorn, whom the *New York Times* dubbed "The Trend Oracle," predicted the cannabis industry would see a corporate feeding frenzy on successful brands similar to the great app boom that began in the tech industry in 2008, though the major players weren't likely to go in big until the United States legalized adult use nationally. Popcorn said corporations such as Kraft weren't likely to start spiking products with THC until they could transport those products across state and international lines.[51]

That day may come sooner than many people think. In April 2018, former Republican speaker of the US House John Boehner, who nine years earlier said he was "unalterably opposed" to cannabis legalization, joined the advisory board of Acreage Holdings, which cultivated, processed, and distributed cannabis in eleven US states. *Fortune* called it a "watershed event" and declared, "Marijuana has gone mainstream."

Former libertarian and Republican Massachusetts governor William Weld, who joined Boehner on the Acreage board—and claimed he had always favored legalization—said he was simply following the times. "Millennials who will inherit the kingdom before long, they are even more positive about cannabis than the populations at large," he said. "You can look at the trend of millennial opinion, and you can see the future."[52]

Or Is Hemp the Future?

As corporate players began to dominate cannabis growing and glut markets, many of the smaller growers who got shut out turned to hemp. In Oregon, where overproduction drove prices as low as $50 per pound, applications for state licenses to grow hemp grew twentyfold from 2015 to 2018.[1]

In 2018, US Republican Senate Majority Leader Mitch McConnell introduced a bill to remove hemp from regulation as a controlled substance and treat it as an agricultural commodity, and analysts predicted hemp products, a $668 million market in 2016, would grow to $2 billion by 2020.

"Hemp is sitting in the background, just waiting to disrupt so many categories when consumer perceptions and legislation change," Susan Gunelius, lead analyst for *Cannabiz Media*, wrote in 2018. "It's an opportunity waiting to be seized."[2]

NOTES

1. Gillian Flaccus, "Marijuana Growers Turning to Hemp as CBD Extract Explodes," AP News, May 14, 2018, https://www.apnews.com/9d36d2784bf94c7684f03b014989e17f/Marijuana-growers-turning-to-hemp-as-CBD-extract-explodes.

2. Susan Gunelius, "Is Hemp the Biggest Opportunity in the Cannabis Market?" *Cannabiz*, February 20, 2018, https://cannabiz.media/hemp-opportunity-cannabis-market/.

Recipes through the Ages

BHANG KI THANDAI, INDIA

Cannabis leaves
Milk
Sugar
Cardamom
Ginger
Melon seeds (optional)

Pound and mix cannabis leaves with water to form a thick paste.

Roll into a ball and let dry.

Mix dried paste with milk, strain through a cloth, mix with more milk or water.

Flavor with sugar, spices such as cardamom and ginger, and sometimes melon seeds.

MAJOUN, INDIA

Bhang goli (bhang paste)
Sesame seed oil
Cocoa butter
Spices
Powdered chocolate
Almonds

Walnuts
Pistachios
Cinnamon
Cloves
Vanilla
Musk
Nutmeg
Belladonna berries
Poppy seeds (optional)
Datura (optional)

Mix together ingredients. Roll into balls.

JATIPHALADI CHURNA, INDIA

Remedy for diarrhea, indigestion, appetite loss, cough, and impotence

Nutmeg
Cinnamon
Ginger
Cumin
Cloves
Cardamom
Pepper
Camphor
Sandalwood
Bamboo manna
Sesame
Tejapatra leaves
Mesua ferrea flowers
Terminalia chebula
T. bellerica
Phyllanthus emblica
Bhang goli (bhang paste)
Sugar

Combine spices, leaves, and flowers. Add bhang goli and sugar. Mix well.

MAJOUN, ISLAMIC

Cannabis leaves
Sesame (optional)
Sugar (optional)

Bake cannabis leaves until they are dry. Rub them between the hands to form a paste. Roll paste into a ball and swallow like a pill.

Alternatively, dry leaves only slightly, then toast and husk them. Mix with sesame and sugar. Chew like gum.

DAWAMESK (ALGERIAN MAJOUN)

Hashish
Sugar
Vanilla
Almonds
Musk
Pistachio
Cinnamon
Orange extract
Cloves
Cardamom
Nutmeg
Cantharides (optional)

Combine all ingredients to make a paste. Roll into balls.

MAJOUN, UNITED STATES

Cannabis resin
Butter
Sugar
Honey
Flour
Henbane

Crushed datura seeds
Opium

Combine all ingredients to form a paste. Shape into lozenges.

FOLK RECIPE, RUSSIA

Hemp seeds
Salt
Bread

Bruise and crush hemp seeds. Roast. Mix with salt.
Spread onto thick slabs of crusty bread.

GUC-KAND, UZBEKISTAN

Hemp leaves and/or flowers
Sugar
Saffron threads
Egg whites

Boil hemp leaves and/or flowers in water until a deep green extract results.

Pour through a strainer. Sweeten the decoction liberally with sugar and add saffron threads and egg whites.

Beat to a frothy paste. Form the mixture into little balls and place in the sun to dry.

Marijuana Medicine by Christian Rätsch, published by Inner Traditions International and Bear & Company, 2001. http://www.Innertraditions.com. Reprinted with permission of the publisher.

JOY PORRIDGE, UZBEKISTAN

Hemp flowers and seeds
Dried leaves
Carnation petals

Pellitory root powder (*Anacyclus pyrethrum*)
Saffron threads
Nutmeg
Cardamom
Almond butter, melted
Honey
Brown sugar

Finely chop all ingredients and add to the melted almond butter.

Add honey and brown sugar and stir to produce a paste.

The dosage must be determined on an individual basis.

HEALTH DRINK OF CANNABIS NECTAR

From Bartolomeo Platina

Cannabis clods
Nard oil

Use a mallet to crush cannabis clods collected after a good harvest.

Add cannabis to nard oil in an iron pot. Crush together over some heat and liquefy.

Carefully treat food and divide for the stomach and the head. Finally, remember everything in excess may be harmful or criminal.

KHYLOS, GREECE

Green cannabis seeds
Water, wine, or mead

Steep green cannabis seeds in water, wine, or mead for "sufficient days" to extract a liquid.

MAJOUN, UNITED STATES

From J. F. Burke, High Times

Hashish
Raw sugar
Powdered arrowroot
Sweet butter
Honey
Cropped, unsalted pistachios

Mix crumbled hashish with raw sugar and powdered arrowroot.

Add sweet butter and mix thoroughly.

Add a little honey and chopped, unsalted pistachios.

"HAPPY SOUP," CAMBODIA

Chicken soup
Cannabis
Lemongrass
Garlic leaf
Chives
Chi ng yeung
Chi bung la

To basic chicken soup, add cannabis, lemongrass, garlic leaf, chives, *chi ng yeung*, and *chi bung la.*

Serve in a ring dish around a small, charcoal chimney.

Glossary of Terms

2-arachidonoylglycerol (2-AG): Endogenous ligand of cannabinoid receptors CB1 and CB2; acts much like CBD.

anandamide: Named after the Sanskrit word for "bliss," an endogenous analogue of tetrahydrocannabinol, similar in structure and function to THC.

Anslinger, Harry J.: As first commissioner of the US Treasury Department's Federal Bureau of Narcotics, from 1930 to 1962, he was largely responsible for cannabis prohibition in the United States. Anslinger was a government civil servant from 1918 to 1963 and served under nine presidents.

Beat generation: Literary movement in 1950s that rejected standard narrative values and materialism.

bhang: Mildly intoxicating preparation of leaves and flowering tops of cannabis made in India.

budtender: A person who sells cannabis at a licensed retail establishment.

butane hash oil (BHO): Extraction made by drawing cannabinoids out of the plant using butane. Known as "honeycomb" or "wax" when it maintains sticky consistency, and "shatter" when it is smooth.

***C. indica*:** Putative species of the genus *Cannabis*, identified by Jean-Baptiste Lamarck.

***C. ruderalis*:** Putative species of the genus *Cannabis*, originally considered a wild breed.

***C. sativa*:** Aromatic annual herbaceous plant indigenous to eastern Asia with palmate leaves and clusters of small, green flowers that can yield tough fibers and act as a euphoriant.

cannabidiol (CBD): A primary cannabinoid in cannabis that doesn't bind to CB1 receptors, where psychoactive effects are triggered, and can mute THC's psychoactive effects.

cannabinoids: Active chemical components in cannabis that plug into cannabinoid receptors in the human brain. Cannabinoids deliver powerful antioxidants and can shift neurological and physiological patterns.

cantharides (Spanish fly): Dangerous, sometimes fatal, mixture of powdered, dried Spanish flies, or blister beetles, sometimes used as a diuretic and aphrodisiac, often added to majoun.

charas: Hashish made from the resin of the cannabis plant in India.

cola: Clusters of female cannabis flowers that can grow up to a foot and more in length.

Cole Memo: US Department of Justice memorandum from US Deputy Attorney General James M. Cole to all US attorneys stating the federal government would not enforce prohibition in states that legalized cannabis, issued on August 29, 2013, and rescinded by Attorney General Jeff Sessions in January 2018.

cultivar: A variety or strain of cannabis originating in and persistent under cultivation.

datura: Shrubby annual plant with large, trumpet-shaped flowers that contains toxic, narcotic alkaloids sometimes used as hallucinogens, often added to majoun.

dawamesk: A spread or jam made in North Africa containing hashish, almond paste, pistachios, sugar, spices, and sometimes cantharides.

decarboxylation: The process of heating cannabis to break off THC-A's and CBD-A's carboxyl radicals, activating THC and CBD and making cannabis more potent.

dispensary: An establishment that sells cannabis. In states where adult-use cannabis is legal, medical dispensaries generally operate separately from "recreational" dispensaries (the cannabis industry prefers the term *adult use*).

distillate: Liquid product made from concentrating, extracting, and isolating cannabinoids and terpenes via steam or fractionation from the cannabis plant.

endocannabinoids: Endogenous lipid-based retrograde neurotransmitters in cannabis plant that bind to cannabinoid receptors in the human body.

extraction: Substance made by extracting cannabinoids from cannabis using a fat or solvent.

extraction artist: A person who is trained and licensed in many techniques to extract and concentrate cannabinoids and terpenes from the cannabis plant.

fan leaf: Large, iconic leaf with long, pointy fingers on the outside of the plant. Fan leaves contain very little THC but, depending on the cultivar, can be high in CBD.

flower: Egg- or conical-shaped cluster of blooms on cannabis plants that grow up to several inches long. Sometimes referred to as *bud* or *nug*.

ganja: Word used for cannabis in India and Jamaica, referring to the Ganges River in India, where cannabis grew freely.

***guc-kand*:** Confection made from cannabis leaves or flowers, sugar, saffron, and egg whites, used to calm crying babies and keep women happy in Uzbekistan.

GW Pharmaceuticals: Global leader in developing cannabinoid-based medicines.

Gysin, Brion: Painter, writer, and performance artist who contributed the Hashish Fudge recipe to *The Alice B. Toklas Cook Book*.

happy pizza: Pizza sprinkled with cannabis, made upon request in Cambodia.

hash: Extracted and concentrated resin from the cannabis plant.

Hassan-ibn-Sabbah: Founder of the *Hashshashin*, a group of assassins, in the eleventh century in northern Persia.

hemp: Nonpsychoactive cannabis subspecies used primarily for food, fiber, and high-CBD medicine.

hippies: A subculture in the 1960s and early 1970s that rejected conventional values and took hallucinogenic drugs.

hydrosol: "Flower water" produced by distilling fresh cannabis leaves, flowers, and other plant material.

infusion: Substance created by extracting chemical compounds from cannabis in a fat or solvent.

kief: Concentrated resin glands that have been separated from the plant using dry, solvent-free methods.

majoun: Moroccan confection made from hashish with any combination of honey, nuts, spices, and dried fruits, sometimes with other drugs such as opium or henbane, that can resemble a candy, paste, or jam.

Marihuana Tax Act of 1937: US act that required every person who sold, dealt, or dispensed cannabis to register with the Internal Revenue Service and pay a special occupational tax, with enforcement provisions for violations of fines of up to $2,000 and five years in prison.

Mechoulam, Raphael: Israeli organic chemist who isolated and identified THC, anandamide, and 2-AG, among other breakthroughs.

phytocannabinoids: Cannabinoids that occur naturally in the cannabis plant.

Pure Food and Drug Act of 1906: Consumer protection law designed to ban foreign and interstate traffic in adulterated or mislabeled food and drug products that included cannabis on a list of dangerous and/or addictive drugs.

shatter: Amber liquid concentrate made using butane.

space cakes: Brownies or cakes made with cannabis, originally available in coffee shops in Amsterdam.

sugar leaf: Small, resin-coated leaves trimmed from colas during harvest, often used in cooking. Also known as *trim*.

tea houses: Speakeasy-type establishments in urban centers that served hashish in the 1920s and 1930s.

terpene: Pungent essential oil produced in cannabis resin that interacts with cannabinoids in the human body to modulate the effects of THC and regulate dopamine and serotonin.

tetrahydrocannabinidinol (THC): Active ingredient in cannabis that gives it psychoactive effects.

tincture: Infusion made by dissolving cannabis in alcohol.

Toklas, Alice B: American-born member of the Parisian avant-garde in the early twentieth century, life partner of writer Gertrude Stein, author of *The Alice B. Toklas Cook Book.*

topical: Cannabis-infused oil, lotion, or balm that is absorbed through the skin for localized relief of pain and inflammation.

trichome: Crystal-like resin gland on cannabis leaves, stems, and calyxes where most cannabinoids and terpenes reside.

UN Single Narcotics Convention of 1961: International treaty to prohibit production and supply of nominally narcotic drugs and drugs with similar effects, regarded as a milestone in the history of international drug control.

wax: Soft, opaque cannabis oils that lose transparency after extraction.

winterization: Using a solvent such as ethanol to remove fats, lipids, and other compounds during the process of extracting cannabinoids and terpenes from cannabis.

Notes

INTRODUCTION

1. "High Times: From Joints to a Lifestyle Movement: The Rise of the Cannabis Economy," J. Walter Thompson Intelligence, 2018, 8.

CHAPTER 1

1. Robert C. Clarke and Mark D. Merlin, *Cannabis: Evolution and Ethnobotany* (Berkeley, CA: University of California Press, 2013), 356.
2. Lucas Laursen, "Botany: The Cultivation of Weed," *Nature*, September 23, 2015, 54.
3. Clarke and Merlin, *Cannabis*, 366.
4. Richard Evans Schultes, William M. Klein, Timothy Plowman, and Tom E. Lockwood, "Cannabis: An Example of Taxonomic Neglect," *Botanical Museum Leaflets, Harvard University* 23, no. 9 (February 28, 1974): 338.
5. Jacob L. Erkelens and Arno Hazekamp, "That Which We Call *Indica*, by Any Other Name Would Smell as Sweet," *Cannabinoids 2014*, 10.
6. Schultes, Klein, Plowman, and Lockwood, "Cannabis," 358.
7. Robert C. Clarke and Mark D. Merlin, "Cannabis Taxonomy: The 'Sativa' vs. 'Indica' Debate," *HerbalGram*, 2016, 45.
8. Ernest Small and Arthur Cronquist, "A Practical and Natural Taxonomy for Cannabis," *Taxon* 25, no. 4 (August 1976): 406.
9. "McPartland's Correct(ed) Vernacular Nomenclature," January 4, 2015, *O'Shaughnessy's Online*.
10. Erkelens and Hazekamp, "That Which We Call *Indica*," 12.

11. John McPartland, "Cannabinoids Involved in Language Acquisition," *O'Shaughnessy's*, Summer 2009, 17.

12. Richard Evans Schultes and Albert Hofmann, *Plants of the Gods: Their Sacred, Healing and Hallucinogenic Powers* (New York: McGraw-Hill, 1979), 10.

13. Clarke and Merlin, *Cannabis*, 212.

14. Carl Sagan, *The Dragons of Eden, Speculations on the Origin of Human Intelligence* (New York: Penguin Books, 1977), 191.

15. Schultes, Klein, Plowman, Lockwood, "Cannabis," 337–38.

16. Clarke and Merlin, *Cannabis*, 51.

17. Barney Warf, "High Points: An Historical Geography of Cannabis," *Geographical Review* 104, no. 4 (2014).

18. Ethan Russo, "Clinical Endocannabinoid Deficiency (CECD): Can This Concept Explain Therapeutic Benefits of Cannabis in Migraine, Fibromyalgia, Irritable Bowel Syndrome and Other Treatment-Resistant Conditions?" *Neuro Endocrinology Letters*, 2008, 199.

19. Pal Pacher, Sandor Batkai, and George Kunos, "The Endocannabinoid System as an Emerging Target of Pharmacotheraphy," *Pharmacological Reviews* 58, no. 3 (2006): 398.

20. Juan Camilo Maldonado Tovar, "Meet the 'Father of Cannabis,' the Man Who Discovered Why Weed Makes You High," Vice.com, February 19, 2016, https://www.vice.com/en_us/article/mvxde4/raphael-mechulam-father-cannabis-discover-thc.

21. "The World's Most Spoken Language Is . . . Terpene," Netherlands Institute of Ecology, 2017, https://nioo.knaw.nl/en/press/worlds-most-spoken-language-isterpene.

22. Ethan B. Russo, "Taming THC: Potential Cannabis Synergy and Phytocannabinoid-Terpenoid Entourage Effects," *British Journal of Pharmacology*, August 2011, 1344–64.

23. Pliny, *Natural History, Books XXIV–XXVII. Vol. 7* (Cambridge, MA: Harvard University Press, 1980), 164.

24. Russo, "Taming THC," 2011.

25. David P. West, "Hemp and Marijuana: Myths & Realities," North American Industrial Hemp Council, 1998, 3, https://www.votehemp.com/PDF/myths_facts.pdf 3.

26. Lester Grinspoon, *Marihuana Reconsidered* (Cambridge, MA: Harvard University Press, 1971), 34.

27. Ernest Small and David Marcus, "Hemp: A New Crop with New Uses for North America," in *Trends in New Crops and New Uses* (Alexandria, VA: ASHA Press, 2002), 284.

28. Eli McVey, "Chart: U.S. Hemp Production Soars in 2017," *Marijuana Business Daily*, March 26, 2018, https://mjbizdaily.com/chart-us-hemp-production-soars-2017/.

29. Morgan Gstalter, "McConnell Bill Would Legalize Hemp as Agricultural Product," *The Hill*, March 26, 2018, http://thehill.com/policy/energy-environment/380287-mcconnell-bill-would-legalize-hemp-as-agricultural-product.

30. Small and Marcus, "Hemp," 294.

31. William Courtney, "Cannabis as a Unique Functional Food," *Treating Yourself* 24, (2010): 54.

32. Courtney, "Cannabis as a Unique Functional Food," 53.

CHAPTER 2

1. Robert C. Clarke and Mark D. Merlin, *Cannabis: Evolution and Ethnobotany* (Berkeley, CA: University of California Press, 2013), 218.

2. Erich Goode, ed., *Marijuana* (Chicago: Atherton, 1969), ix.

3. Clark and Merlin, *Cannabis*, 204.

4. Mia Touw, "The Religious and Medicinal Uses of *Cannabis* in China, India and Tibet," *Journal of Psychoactive Drugs* 13, no. 1 (January–March 1981), https://www.cnsproductions.com/pdf/Touw.pdf.

5. Clarke and Merlin, *Cannabis*.

6. Ethan B. Russo, Hong-En Jiang, Xiao Li, Alan Sutton, et al., "Phytochemical and Genetic Analyses of Ancient Cannabis from Central Asia," *Journal of Experimental Botany* 59, no. 15 (November 2008): 4171–82, https://www.ncbi.nlm.nih.gov/pmc/articles/PMC2639026/.

7. Barney Warf, "High Points: An Historical Geography of Cannabis," *Geographical Review* 104, no. 4 (2014), http://www.questia.com/read/1G1-387952804/high-points-an-historical-geography-of-cannabis.

8. E. L. Abel, *Marihuana: The First Twelve Thousand Years* (New York: Springer Publishing, 1980), 18.

9. Lester Grinspoon, *Marihuana Reconsidered* (Cambridge, MA: Harvard University Press, 1971), 40.

10. Grinspoon, *Marihuana Reconsidered*, 40–41.

11. Touw, "The Religious and Medicinal Uses of *Cannabis*," 4.

12. Tod Mikuriya, "Introduction to the Indian Hemp Drugs Commission Report," Comitas Institute for Anthropological Study, http://cifas.us/analyses/Mikuriya1.html.

13. Isaac Campos, *Home Grown: Marijuana and the Origins of Mexico's War on Drugs* (Chapel Hill, NC: University of North Carolina Press, 2012), 9.

14. Campos, *Home Grown*, 14.

15. Mikuriya, "Introduction to the Indian Hemp Drugs Commission Report."

16. Gertrude Emerson Sen, *Voiceless India*, revised ed. (New York: John Day Company, 1944), 196.

17. Raphael Mechoulam, *Cannabinoids as Therapeutics* (New York: Springer Science & Business Media, 2006), 17.

18. Daphna Hacker, "Colonialism's Civilizing Mission: The Case of the Indian Hemp Drugs Commission," Tel Aviv University, 2001, 458, http://law.bepress.com/cgi/viewcontent.cgi?article=1161&context=taulwps.

19. "Report of the Indian Hemp Drugs Commission, 1893–94," 15, https://digital.nls.uk/indiapapers/browse/archive/74464868.

20. "Report of Indian Hemp Drugs Commission," 16.

21. Grinspoon, *Marihuana Reconsidered*, 173.

22. David L. Haberman, *Journey through the Twelve Forests: An Encounter with Krishna* (New York: Oxford University Press, 1994), 212.

23. Haberman, *Journey through the Twelve Forests*, 47.

24. Richard Connerney, *The Upside-Down Tree: India's Changing Culture* (New York: Algora, 2009), 101–2.

25. Dean Latimer, "Hashish and Terrorism," *High Times*, July 1978, 52.

26. Clark and Merlin, *Cannabis*, 232.

27. Abel, *Marihuana*, 22.

28. Campos, *Home Grown*, 11.

29. Clarke and Merlin, *Cannabis*, 234.

30. Campos, *Home Grown*, 13.

31. Isaac Littlebury, *The History of Herodotus, 1737* (London: Kessinger Publishing, 2010), 380.

32. Warf, "High Points," 104.

33. Clarke and Merlin, *Cannabis*, 206.

34. Vera Rubin (ed.), *Cannabis and Culture* (The Hague: Mouton Publishers, 1975), 39–49.

35. Christian Rätsch, *Marijuana Medicine: A World Tour of the Healing and Visionary Powers of Cannabis* (Rochester, VT: Healing Arts Press, 2001), 122.

36. Benjamin Kemper, "The Quest for an Ancient Culture's Cannabis-Filled Cooking," *Atlas Obscura*, May 2, 2018, https://www.atlasobscura.com/articles/cannabis-cooking-in-georgia?utm_source=Gastro+Obscura+Weekly+E-mail&utm_campaign=2f03b5df80-EMAIL_CAMPAIGN_2018_05_07&utm_medium=email&utm_term=0_2418498528-2f03b5df80-68458689&mc_cid=2f03b5df80&mc_eid=b6753bc786.

37. George Nelson, "Georgia Eases Draconian Law on Cannabis Use," *The Guardian*, January 24, 2017, https://www.theguardian.com/world/2017/jan/24/georgia-eases-draconian-law-cannabis-landmark-ruling.

38. Rubin, *Cannabis and Culture*, 42.

39. Clarke and Merlin, *Cannabis*, 233.

40. Russo et al., "Phytochemical and Genetic Analyses," 36.

41. Ethan B. Russo and Franjo Grotenhermen, *The Handbook of Cannabis Therapeutics: From Bench to Bedside* (Binghamton, NY: The Haworth Press, 2006), 26.

42. Richard Rose, "It's Nigh Time to Grandfather Hemp," Hemp.com, May 31, 2018, http://www.hemp.com/2018/05/its-nigh-time-to-grandfather-hemp/.

43. Robert Deitch, *Hemp: American History Revisited—The Plant with a Divided History* (New York: Algora, 2003), 46.

CHAPTER 3

1. Isaac Campos, *Home Grown: Marijuana and the Origins of Mexico's War on Drugs* (Chapel Hill, NC: University of North Carolina Press, 2012), 14–15.

2. Ethan B. Russo and Franjo Grotenhermen, *Handbook of Cannabis Therapeutics: From Bench to Bedside* (Binghamton, NY: The Haworth Press, 2006), 14.

3. Lester Grinspoon, *Marihuana Reconsidered* (Cambridge, MA: Harvard University Press, 1971), 58.

4. Grinspoon, *Marihuana Reconsidered*, 59–62.

5. Grinspoon, *Marihuana Reconsidered*, 55–58.

6. Lester Grinspoon, "Opium, Not Alcohol, Is the Demon," *New York Times*, October 24, 1971, 58.

7. Charles Baudelaire, "The Poem of Hashish," Erowid.org, https://www.erowid.org/culture/characters/baudelaire_charles/baudelaire_charles_poem1.shtml.

8. Alexandre Dumas, *The Count of Monte Cristo* (London: Chapman and Hall, 1844), 539.

9. Bayard Taylor, *The Lands of the Saracen* (New York: G. P. Putnam, 1863), http://www.gutenberg.org/files/10924/10924-h/10924-h.htm#ch10.

10. Fitz Hugh Ludlow, *The Hasheesh Eater: Being Passages from the Life of a Pythagorean* (Calgary, Alberta: Theophania Publishing, 2011), xi; Amy Roach, "Fitz Hugh Ludlow, Hasheesh Eater," *Potent*, https://potent.media/fitz-hugh-ludlow-hasheesh-eater.

11. H. H. Kane, "A Hashish-House in New York," *Harper's* 667 (November 1883): 944–49.

12. Kane, "A Hashish-House in New York."

13. Glenn O'Brien and Gary Stimeling, "Interview: Vera Rubin," *High Times*, June 1978, 33.

14. Jon Bradshaw, "The Reggae Way to 'Salvation,'" *New York Times*, August 14, 1977, 183.

15. Leonard Barrett Sr., *The Rastafarians* (Boston, MA: Beacon Press, 1997), 2.

16. Stephen Davis, "Fear in Paradise," *New York Times*, July 25, 1976, 153.

17. Barrett, *The Rastafarians*, 141.

18. Pamela Lloyd, "1974: A Century of Reefer Action in Five Years; or, Time Flies When You're Having Fun," *High Times*, 56.

19. Vera D. Rubin, *Ganja in Jamaica: A Medical Anthropological Study of Chronic Marihuana Use* (The Hague: Moutaon De Gruyter), 26.

20. Davidacus Holmes, "The Rasta Lifestyle, Ital Food, Ganja Farming in Jamaica, Ganja as Sacrament," Filmed February 2015, YouTube video, Posted June 2017, https://www.youtube.com/watch?v=FI1tmqhOHwE.

21. Adrian Frater, "No to Edible Ganja Products—Ras Iyah V . . . Calls for Cannabis-Oriented Educational Programmes," *Jamaica Gleaner*, May 31, 2017, http://jamaica-gleaner.com/article/lead-stories/20170531/no-edible-ganja-products-ras-iyah-v-calls-cannabis-oriented.

22. Jack Herer, *The Emperor Wears No Clothes: Hemp and the Marijuana Conspiracy* (Van Nuys, CA: Ah Ha Publishing, 1985), 160.

23. Campos, *Home Grown*, 206.

24. Campos, *Home Grown*, 3.

25. Campos, *Home Grown*, 204.

26. Herer, *The Emperor Wears No Clothes*, 299.

27. Barney Warf, "High Points: An Historical Geography of Cannabis," *Geographical Review* 104, no. 4 (2014).

28. Warf, "High Points."

29. *Mail Order Drug Paraphernalia Control Act, Hearing Before the Subcommittee on Crime of the Committee on the Judiciary, House of Representatives, Ninety-Ninth Congress, Second Session on H.R. 1625, May 8, 1986* (ReInk Books, 2017), 121.

30. "Use of Marijuana Spreading in West, Poisonous Weed Is Being Sold Quite Freely in Pool Halls and Beer Gardens. Children Said to Buy It, Narcotic Bureau Officials Say Law Gives No Authority to Stop Traffic," *New York Times*, September 16, 1934, 6.

31. Harry Jacob Anslinger, *Marijuana: Assassin of Youth* (New York: Crowell Publishing, 1937), https://www.redhousebooks.com/galleries/assassin.htm.

32. Ernest L. Abel, *Marihuana: The First Twelve Thousand Years* (New York: Springer Publishing, 1980), 224.

33. Anslinger, *Marijuana*.

34. Herer, *The Emperor Wears No Clothes*.

35. Grinspoon, *Marihuana Reconsidered*, 21.

36. Robert Deitch, *Hemp: American History Revisited—the Plant with a Divided History* (New York: Algora, 2003), 147.

37. "Drive on Narcotics Sped by Treasury; Campaign to Rid the Nation of Marijuana Is a Feature of Year's Program," *New York Times*, January 31, 1938, 12.

38. Joel Fort, "Pot: A Rational Approach," *Playboy*, October 1969, 130.

39. Dan Baum, "Legalize It All," *Harper's*, April 2016, https://harpers.org/archive/2016/04/legalize-it-all/.

40. Chris Bennett, "The Incredible, Delectable, Miracle of 19th Century Medicine: Hasheesh Candy!" *Cannabis Culture*, February 7, 2013, https://www.cannabisculture.com/content/2013/02/07/incredible-delectable-miracle-19th-century-medicine-hasheesh-candy.

41. Dale Gieringer, "A Warning Re Dabs," *O'Shaughnessy's* Online, http://www.beyondthc.com/a-warning-re-dabs/.

CHAPTER 4

1. Belinda Bruner, "A Recipe for Modernism and the Somatic Intellect in the *Alice B. Toklas Cook Book* and Gertrude Stein's 'Tender Buttons,'" *Papers on Language & Literature* 45, no. 4 (2009): 411.

2. John Geiger, *Nothing Is True, Everything Is Permitted: The Life of Brion Gysin* (New York: Disinformation Books, 2005), 106.

3. "Alice B. Toklas Reads Her Famous Recipe for Hashish Fudge," *Open Culture*, January 22, 2014, http://www.openculture.com/2014/01/alice-b-toklas-talks-about-her-famous-recipe-for-hashish-fudge.html.

4. Geiger, *Nothing Is True*, 107.

5. Geiger, *Nothing Is True*, 107.

6. "Life Guide," *Life*, September 29, 1961, 28.

7. Geiger, *Nothing Is True*, 106.

8. "Alice Toklas, 89, Is Dead in Paris," *New York Times*, March 8, 1967, https://archive.nytimes.com/www.nytimes.com/books/98/05/03/specials/stein-toklasobit.html?_r=1&oref=slogin.

9. John Birdsall, "Jeremiah Tower's Invincible Armor of Pleasure," *Eater*, November 7, 2014, https://www.eater.com/2014/11/7/7166097/jeremiah-towers-invincible-armor-of-pleasure.

10. Dan Wakefield, "The Prodigal Powers of Pot: Acclaimed by Ancients, Frowned on by Fuzz, Beatified by Beats, Marijuana Remains the Most Misunderstood Drug of All Time," *Playboy*, August 1962, 52.

11. Dwight Garner, "Trusting in *The Sheltering Sky*, Even When It Scorched," *New York Times*, August 30, 2009, https://www.nytimes.com/2009/08/31/books/31bowles.html.

12. Layla Eplett, "Go Ask Alice: The History of Toklas' Legendary Hashish Fudge," *Scientific American*, April 20, 2015, https://blogs.scientificamerican.com/food-matters/go-ask-alice-the-history-of-toklas-8217-legendary-hashish-fudge/.

13. Paul O'Neil, "The Only Rebellion Around, But the Shabby Beats Bungle the Job in Arguing, Sulking and Bad Poetry," *Life*, November 30, 1959, 115.

14. Ira Cohen, "The Goblet of Dreams," *Playboy*, April 1966, 125–28.

15. Timothy Leary, "Majoon and the Mind," *Playboy*, July 1966, 16.

16. Lester Grinspoon, *Marihuana Reconsidered* (Cambridge, MA: Harvard University Press, 1971), 202.

17. Roger Vaughan, "Mad New Scene on Sunset, Strip," *Life*, August 26, 1966, 75.

18. Barry Farrell, "The Other Culture: An Explorer of the Worldwide Underground of Art Finds, Behind Its Orgiastic Happenings, Brutalities and Pot-Seed Pancakes, a Wild Utopian Dream," *Life*, February 17, 1967, 87.

19. "Marijuana: Millions of Turned-On Users," *Life*, July 7, 1967, 21.

20. Roger Ebert, *The Great Movies IV* (Chicago: University of Chicago Press, 2016), 248.

21. Roger Ebert, "I Love You, Alice B. Toklas," November 27, 1968, https://www.rogerebert.com/reviews/i-love-you-alice-b-toklas-1968.

22. "I Love You, Alice B. Toklas!" *Variety*, December 31, 1967, http://variety.com/1967/film/reviews/i-love-you-alice-b-toklas-1200421625/.

23. Vincent Canby, "Screen: 'I Love You, Alice B. Toklas!'" *New York Times*, October 8, 1968, https://timesmachine.nytimes.com/timesmachine/1968/10/08/76888012.pdf.

24. Geiger, *Nothing Is True*, 224.

25. P. J. Geerlings, "Treatment of Drug Addicts," *Maandblad voor Geestelijke Volksgezondheid* 30, no. 11 (1975): 49–52, 51.

26. "Coffee Shops in Amsterdam: Why Are the Amsterdam Cannabis Cafes Allowed?" http://www.amsterdam-advisor.com/coffee-shops-in-amsterdam.html.

27. Barney Warf, "High Points: An Historical Geography of Cannabis," *Geographical Review* 104, no. 4 (2014), http://www.questia.com/read/1G1-387952804/high-points-an-historical-geography-of-cannabis.

28. Reg Potterton, "Amsterdam . . . " *Playboy*, March 1971, 135.

29. "Hooray! The Bulldog Turned 40 in 2015!" https://www.thebulldog.com/40-years-the-living-room-of-amsterdam/.

30. Simon Vinkenoog, "Dutch Beat," *High Times*, June 1986, 53.

31. "'Low-Risk' Drug Sales Considered Acceptable: In Amsterdam, Cannabis Is High on Coffee Shop Menu," *Los Angeles Times*, November 2, 1986, http://articles.latimes.com/1986-11-02/news/mn-15818_1_coffee-shop.

32. Jenna Valleriani, "On Dutch Coffeeshops and Vancouver Dispensaries," *Lift*, January 13, 2016, https://news.lift.co/dutch-coffeeshops-canada-dispensaries/.

33. T. Alan Schack, "Report from Amsterdam: The New Breed of Coffeeshops," *High Times*, November 1994, 11.

34. Shane Blackman, *Chilling Out: The Cultural Politics of Substance Consumption, Youth and Drug Policy* (Maidenhead, England: Open University Press, 2003), 177.

35. Michael Pollan, "How Pot Has Grown," *New York Times Magazine*, February 18, 1995, https://www.nytimes.com/1995/02/19/magazine/how-pot-has-grown.html.

36. A. C. M. Jansen, "The Economics of Cannabis-Cultivation in Europe," paper presented at the 2nd European Conference on Drug Trafficking and Law Enforcement. Paris, September 26 and 27, 2002, http://www.cedro-uva.org/lib/jansen.economics.html.

37. Robert J. MacCoun and Peter Reuter, *Drug War Heresies: Learning from Other Vices, Times, and Places* (Cambridge, England: Cambridge University Press, 2001), 241.

38. Robert J. MacCoun, "What Can We Learn from the Dutch Cannabis Coffeeshop System?" Goldman School of Public Policy and UC Berkeley School of Law, University of California, Berkeley, CA, October 22, 2010, http://gspp.berkeley.edu/assets/uploads/research/pdf/MacCoun2011_Dutch-CannabisCoffeeshopSystem.pdf.

39. Gavin Haines, "Why Amsterdam's Oldest Cannabis 'Coffeeshop' Has Been Forced to Close," *Telegraph*, January 3, 2017, https://www.telegraph.co.uk/travel/destinations/europe/netherlands/amsterdam/articles/amsterdams-oldest-coffeeshop-mellow-yellow-is-forced-to-close/.

40. Atossa Araxia Abrahamian, "Baking Bad: A Potted History of 'High Times,'" *The Nation*, October 30, 2013, https://www.thenation.com/article/baking-bad-potted-history-high-times/.

41. J. F. Burke, "Eat It!" *High Times*, February 1978, 47–49.

42. Mike Gianakos, "500 Issues of *High Times*: A History of the World's Most Notorious Magazine," HighTimes.com, August 30, 2017, https://hightimes.com/culture/500-issues-of-high-times-a-history-of-the-worlds-most-notorious-magazine/.

43. "That First Joint," by Chef Ra, *High Times*, November 2007, 20.

44. "The *High Times* Interview: Action Bronson," by Elise McDonough, *High Times*, July 2016, 104.

45. Daniel Victor, "*High Times* Is Sold to Group That Includes Son of Bob Marley," *New York Times*, June 1, 2017, https://www.nytimes.com/2017/06/01/business/media/high-times-magazine-marijuana.html.

46. Peter Gorman, "Cambodia: Where Marijuana Is Legal," *High Times*, September 1994, 49.

47. Ethan Harfenist and Bennett Murray, "The High Life," *Phnom Penh Post*, May 29, 2015, https://www.phnompenhpost.com/post-weekend/high-life.

48. Sudough Nimn, "Khmer Green: The Happy Herb," *High Times*, September 1999, 65.

49. "Tony Bourdain—HAPPY PIZZA!!!!" YouTube video, 1:26, posted by Desiree West, March 8, 2011, https://www.youtube.com/watch?time_continue=81&v=8t2kvMIi8h0.

50. Max Winkler, "Phnom Penh's Happy Pizza Left Me High and Dry," *Vice*, September 29, 2017, https://munchies.vice.com/en_us/article/mgxywp/phnom-penhs-happy-pizza-left-me-high-and-dry.

51. Jen Polachek, "Getting Buzzed: Cooking with Pot," *Huffington Post*, December 6, 2017, https://www.huffingtonpost.com/saveur/cooking-with-pot_b_927648.html.

52. Dania Putri and Tom Blickman, "Cannabis in Indonesia: Patterns in Consumption, Production, and Policies," Transnational Institute, January 2016, https://www.tni.org/filtion-downloads/dpb_44_13012016_map_web.pdfes/publica.

53. Meagan Angus, "Remembering the Florence Nightingale of Medical Marijuana," *Seattle Weekly*, June 29, 2016, http://www.seattleweekly.com/food/remembering-the-florence-nightingale-of-medical-marijuana/.

54. "Cops Pop 'Brownie Mary,'" *High Times*, May 1981, 2.

55. Carey Goldberg, "Brownie Mary Fights to Legalize Marijuana," *New York Times*, July 6, 1996, https://www.nytimes.com/1996/07/06/us/brownie-mary-fights-to-legalize-marijuana.html.

56. Albin Krebs and Robert M. C. G. Thomas, "Notes on People; Alice B. Toklas Goodies," *New York Times*, Saturday, January 17, 1981, https://www.nytimes.com/1981/01/17/nyregion/notes-on-people-alice-b-toklas-goodies.html.

57. Peter Gorman, "Interview: Brownie Mary Rathburn," *High Times*, January 1993, 50.

58. Gorman, "Interview," 51.

59. Peter Gorman, "Brownie Mary Busted: Faces Five Years for Baking Magic Brownies for PWAs," December 1992, 23.

60. Gorman, "Interview," 50.

61. Christopher Reed, "'Brownie Mary' Rathbun," *The Guardian*, May 19, 1999, https://www.theguardian.com/news/1999/may/20/guardianobituaries1.

62. Peter Hecht, *Weed Land: Inside America's Marijuana Epicenter and How Pot Went Legit* (Oakland: University of California Press, 2014), 49.

63. Carey Goldberg, "Marijuana Club Helps Those in Pain," *New York Times*, February 25, 1996, https://www.nytimes.com/1996/02/25/us/marijuana-club-helps-those-in-pain.html.

64. Goldberg, "Marijuana Club Helps Those in Pain."

65. Trina Robbins, "Brownie Mary: Good-Bye to a Saint," *High Times*, August 1, 1999, 22.

CHAPTER 5

1. Patricia King and Marc Peyser, "Pot Shots in the War on Drugs: 'Doonesbury' Mixes It Up over Marijuana," *Newsweek*, October 14, 1996, 12.

2. Peter Gorman, "Feds Fly Anti-Pot Doc Balloon," *High Times*, April 1997, 20.

3. Duchess of York Sarah, "The Battle for Medical Marijuana," *The Nation*, January 6, 1997, http://www.questia.com/read/1G1-18994067/the-battle-for-medical-marijuana.

4. Nick Gillespie, "Prescription: Drugs," *Reason*, February 1997, http://www.questia.com/read/1G1-19192456/prescription-drugs.

5. Christopher S. Wren, "Votes on Marijuana Are Stirring Debate," *New York Times*, November 17, 1996, https://www.nytimes.com/1996/11/17/us/votes-on-marijuana-are-stirring-debate.html.

6. "Waiting to Inhale Customers Pack Marijuana Store Reopening after U.S. Raid," *St. Louis Post-Dispatch (MO)*, January 16, 1997, http://www.questia.com/read/1P2-33047729/waiting-to-inhale-customers-pack-marijuana-store-reopening.

7. Dr. Lester Grinspoon, "Cannabis Clubs: Public Nuisance or Therapy?" *Playboy*, November 1998, 44.

8. Michael Pollan, "Living with Medical Marijuana," *New York Times*, July 28, 1997, https://www.nytimes.com/1997/07/20/magazine/living-with-medical-marijuana.html.

9. David Samuels, "Dr. Kush," *The New Yorker*, July 28, 2008, http://www.questia.com/read/1P3-1520182561/dr-kush.

10. Peter Hecht, *Weed Land: Inside America's Marijuana Epicenter and How Pot Went Legit* (Oakland: University of California Press, 2014), 5.

11. Hecht, *Weed Land*, 24.

12. "Stories of Amendment 64 Oral History Project," Mason Tvert, interviewed by Janet Bishop (Colorado State Library), https://dspace.library.colostate.edu/bitstream/handle/10217/176472/AMNT_OralHistoryTranscript_Tverk-part3.pdf?sequence=3&isAllowed=y.

13. "Stories of Amendment 64 Oral History Project," Jeanna Hoch, interviewed by Janet Bishop (Colorado State Library), https://dspace.library.colostate.edu/handle/10217/176470.

14. "Stories of Amendment 64 Oral History Project," Christian Sederberg, interviewed by Janet Bishop (Colorado State Library), https://dspace.library.colostate.edu/bitstream/handle/10217/176469/AMNT_OralHistoryTranscript_Sederberg-part2-sect2.pdf?sequence=11&isAllowed=y.

15. Sederberg interview.

16. Chandra Thomas Whitfield, "Capitalizing on Cannabis: Meet Colorado's Black 'Potrepreneurs,'" NBCNews.com, April 19, 2015, https://www.nbcnews.com/news/nbcblk/capitalizing-cannabis-meet-colorado-s-black-potrepreneurs-n344556.

17. David Bienenstock, "Cannabis Edibles That Changed the Game," *Leafly*, February 22, 2018, https://www.leafly.com/news/strains-products/7-weed-edibles-that-changed-the-game.

18. Maureen Dowd, "Don't Harsh Our Mellow, Dude," *New York Times,* June 3, 2014, https://www.nytimes.com/2014/06/04/opinion/dowd-dont-harsh-our-mellow-dude.html.

19. Bruce Barcott, "The Great Marijuana Experiment: A Tale of Two Drug Wars," *Rolling Stone*, January 3, 2014, https://www.rollingstone.com/politics/news/the-great-marijuana-experiment-a-tale-of-two-drug-wars-20140103.

20. Alicia Wallace, "Colorado Marijuana Sales Hit $1.5 Billion in 2017," *The Cannabist*, February 9, 2018, https://www.thecannabist.co/2018/02/09/colorado-rijuana-sales-december-year-2017/98606/.

21. Elise McDonough, "California's Cannabis Edibles Just Got Surprisingly Boring," *Vice Munchies*, January 8, 2018, https://munchies.vice.com/en_us/article/3k55qj/californias-cannabis-edibles-just-got-surprisingly-boring.

22. Robyn Griggs Lawrence, "Is Cannabis Chocolate the Ultimate Edible?" *High Times*, February 13, 2017, https://hightimes.com/edibles/is-cannabis-chocolate-the-ultimate-edible/.

23. Lawrence, "Is Cannabis Chocolate the Ultimate Edible?"

24. Lawrence, "Is Cannabis Chocolate the Ultimate Edible?"

25. Robyn Griggs Lawrence, "Terpene and Turn On!" *Sensi*, January 29, 2018, http://www.sensimag.com/2018/01/29/165814/terpene-and-turn-on.

26. Robyn Griggs Lawrence, "Just Add Water," *Sensi*, Boulder/Denver edition, February 2018, 88.

27. Lawrence, "Just Add Water," 88.

28. Lori Jane Gliha and Serene Fang, "Colorado Cannabis Czar: We Didn't Anticipate Problems with Pot Edibles," *Al Jazeera*, January 7, 2015, http://america.aljazeera.com/watch/shows/america-tonight/articles/2015/1/7/colorado-cannabisczarwedidntanticipateproblemswithpotedibles.html.

29. "Vermonters Visit to Colorado to Study Legalized Marijuana," 10, https://legislature.vermont.gov/assets/Documents/2016/WorkGroups/House%20Judiciary/Reports%20and%20Resources/W~Department%20of%20Public%20Safety~Vermonters%20Visit%20to%20Colorado%20to%20Study%20Legalized%20Marijuana~3-11-2015.pdf.

30. Jack Healy, "New Scrutiny on Sweets with Ascent of Marijuana in Colorado," *New York Times*, October 29, 2014, https://www.nytimes.com/2014/10/30/us/new-scrutiny-on-sweets-with-ascent-of-marijuana-in-colorado.html.

31. D. G. Barrus, K. L. Capogrossi, S. C. Cates, et al., "Tasty THC: Promises and Challenges of Cannabis Edibles," *Methods Report (RTI Press)*, November 2016, https://www.ncbi.nlm.nih.gov/pmc/articles/PMC5260817/.

32. Robert J. MacCoun and Michelle M. Mello, "Half-Baked—The Retail Promotion of Marijuana Edibles," *New England Journal of Medicine*, March 12, 2015, https://www.nejm.org/doi/full/10.1056/NEJMp1416014.

33. Ricardo Oliveira, "The Promises and Challenges of Cannabis Edibles," *Lift*, February 6, 2017, https://news.lift.co/promises-challenges-cannabis-edibles/.

34. Joshua Miller, "Colorado Serves Edible Marijuana with a Side of Controversy," *Boston Globe*, September 16, 2016, https://www.hfcm.org/CMS/Images/Boston%20Globe.Colorado%20serves%20edible%20marijuana%20with%20a%20side%20of%20controversy.9.16.16.pdf.

35. Courtney Flatt, "Can the Cannabis Industry Deliver an Organic, Environmentally Sensitive High?" OPB.org, December 23, 2016, https://www.opb.org/news/article/organically-grown-marijuana/.

36. Jack Kaskey, "Pot Laced with Pesticides Forces States to Act as EPA Stays Away," *Bloomberg*, August 2, 2017, https://www.bloomberg.com/news/articles/2017-08-02/pot-laced-with-pesticides-forces-states-to-act-as-epa-stays-away.

37. Joe Klare, "Legal Pot's Pesticide Problem: What Can Be Done About It," *Marijuana Times*, March 24, 2017, https://www.marijuanatimes.org/legal-pots-pesticide-problem-what-can-be-done-about-it/.

38. "Colorado Cannabis and the Use of Pesticides: Where Are We At?" *The Cannabist*, May 19, 2016, https://www.thecannabist.co/2016/05/19/colorado-cannabis-pesticides-update/54430/.

39. Amanda Pampuro, "Talk About Pot Luck! Ganja Gourmet Gets Ready for Its Next Course," *Westword*, April 19, 2017, http://www.westword.com/marijuana/ganja-gourmet-prepares-for-the-next-step-in-the-edible-evolution-8985358.

40. Lauren Viera, "Better Than Pot Brownies, by a James Beard Award–Winning Chef," *Times Style Magazine*, March 24, 2016, https://www.nytimes.com/2016/03/24/t-magazine/marijuana-chocolate-candy-mindy-segal.html.

41. Jesse Pearson, "Weed and Stoner Food, Together at Last," *GQ*, July 2, 2012, http://www.gq.com/story/weed-and-stoner-food-recipes-robertas-brooklyn.

42. Jesse Hirsch, "Local Cannabis Chefs Are Out to Prove Their Dinners Can Be More Than Dope," *Edible Brooklyn*, March 23, 2017, https://www.ediblebrooklyn.com/2017/local-cannabis-chefs-prove-dinners-more-dope/.

43. Beca Grimm, "Baked to Perfection: This Stoned Scone Goes Perfectly with Your 'Tea' HC," *Merry Jane*, August 9, 2017, https://merryjane.com/culture/baked-to-perfection-jessica-coles-date-scones-white-rabbit-high-tea.

44. Andy Wright, "Beyond Brownies: The Science of Cooking with Cannabis," *Splendid Table*, May 4, 2017, https://www.splendidtable.org/story/beyond-brownies-the-science-of-cooking-with-cannabis.

45. Chris Sayegh, "The Herbal Chef on Terpenes: Chris Sayegh Breaks Down These Fragrant, Flavorful Oils," *Dope*, July 30, 2017, http://www.dopemagazine.com/herbal-chef-terpenes-chris-sayegh-breaks-fragrant-flavorful-oils/.

46. Steve Baltin, "Meet the Herbal Chef, the Man Turning Weed-Infused Food Gourmet," *Forbes*, December 5, 2017, https://www.forbes.com/sites/stevebaltin/2017/12/05/meet-the-herbal-chef-the-man-turning-weed-infused-food-gourmet/#248058c5b246.

47. Marcia Gagliardi, "Underground Cannabis Dinners Are Creating Quite a Buzz in the Bay Area (and Wine Is No Longer the Primary Food Pairing)," KQED.org, December 29, 2017, https://www.kqed.org/bayareabites/124226/underground-cannabis-dinners-are-creating-quite-a-buzz-in-the-bay-area-and-wine-is-no-longer-the-primary-food-pairing.

48. Ed Murrieta, "America's Top 10 Cannabis Chefs," *GreenState*, November 22, 2017, http://www.greenstate.com/food-travel/americas-top-10-cannabis-chefs/.

49. Jackie Bryant, "San Diego Pop-Up Dinners Pair Cannabis with Food," *Eater San Diego*, February 14, 2018, https://sandiego.eater.com/2018/2/14/17011216/san-diego-cannabis-marijuana-dinners.

50. Christina Orlovsky Page, "Cannabis Dinners Are Becoming 'Almost Socially Acceptable,'" *San Diego Magazine*, August 1, 2017, http://www.sandiegomagazine.com/San-Diego-Magazine/August-2017/Cannabis-Dinners-are-Becoming-Almost-Socially-Acceptable/.

51. Mike Sula, "Herbal Notes Is Planting the Seeds of Culinary Cannabis in Chicago," *Chicago Reader*, https://www.chicagoreader.com/chicago/herbal-notes-culinary-cannabis-weed-dinners-manny-mendoza/Content?oid=45808759.

52. Danya Henninger, "David Ansill's Next Act: Marijuana-Infused Pop-Up Dinners," *Billypenn*, January 29, 2017, https://billypenn.com/2017/01/29/david-ansills-next-act-marijuana-infused-pop-up-dinners/.

53. Hannah Goldfield, "A Marijuana Dinner Party Grows Underground," *The New Yorker*, March 8, 2018, https://www.newyorker.com/culture/tables-for-two/an-underground-marijuana-dinner-party-grows-in-new-york?mbid=social_facebook.

54. David Jenison, "Meet the Duo Behind NYC's Hottest Cannabis Speakeasies," Prohibtd.com, https://prohbtd.com/meet-the-duo-behind-nycs-hottest-cannabis-speakeasies.

55. Lars Himmerskov Eriksen, "Cooking with Cannabis—a New Culinary High?" *The Guardian*, January 7, 2014, https://www.theguardian.com/lifeandstyle/wordofmouth/2014/jan/07/cooking-cannabis-culinary-high-novelty-ingredient-hemp-chefs.

56. Jorges Cervantes, "The Reign of Spain: A Festive Mediterranean Lifestyle and Favorable Laws Have Made Spain the New Cannabis Capital of Europe," *High Times*, June 2004, 31.

57. Maureen Meehan, "Has Spain Become Europe's Marijuana Garden? Experts Say Si," *High Times*, June 20, 2017, https://hightimes.com/news/has-spain-become-europes-marijuana-garden-experts-say-si/.

58. Rick Steves, "Want to Smoke Marijuana in Spain? Join a Club," *Huffington Post*, May 24, 2016, https://www.huffingtonpost.com/rick-steves/want-to-smoke-marijuana-i_b_10121928.html.

59. Danny Danko, "Spain," *High Times*, December 2013, 50.

60. Malia Politzer, "Barcelona's Pot Boom and Bust: The Uncertain Fate of Cannabis Clubs in 'The Amsterdam of Southern Europe,'" *Reason*, March 2016, http://www.questia.com/read/1G1-443399249/barcelona-s-pot-boom-and-bust-the-uncertain-fate.

61. "Code of Conduct for European Cannabis Social Clubs," December 9, 2011, http://www.encod.org/info/CODE-OF-CONDUCT-FOR-EUROPEAN.html.

62. Stoney Xochi, "Reflections from Barcelona: Spannabis 2017," *Cannabis Now*, March 28, 2017, https://cannabisnow.com/reflections-barcelona-spannabis-2017/.

63. Beth McGroarty, "2015 Trends Report," *Spafinder Wellness 365*, 2015, 15.

64. Valerie Labonne, "The Booming Business of Cannabis in Spain," *France 24*, April 29, 2017, http://www.france24.com/en/20170428-reporters-spain-cannabis-clubs-marijuana-tourism-business-economy-illegal-production.

65. Uki Goni, "High Times in Montevideo: Uruguay Entering Brave New World of Pot Legalization," *Time*, August 5, 2013, http://world.time.com/2013/08/05/high-times-in-montevideo-uruguay-enters-brave-new-world-of-pot-legalization/.

66. Mariela Murdocco, "Uruguay: The World's Laboratory for Marijuana Legalisation," *The Guardian*, October 4, 2013, https://www.theguardian.com/commentisfree/2013/oct/04/uruguay-legalize-marijuana-george-soros.

67. John Walsh and Geoff Ramsey, "Uruguay's Drug Policy: Major Innovations, Major Challenges," Foreign Policy at Brookings, 2016, https://www.brookings.edu/wp-content/uploads/2016/07/Walsh-Uruguay-final.pdf.

68. Madison Margolin, "Weed's Legal in Uruguay, But It Looks Nothing Like Colorado," *Jane Street*, July 11, 2017, https://janest.com/article/2017/07/11/weeds-legal-uruguay-looks-nothing-like-colorado/.

69. Leonardo Haberkorn, "'Gourmet Cannabis': Take a Peek Inside a Uruguay Marijuana Club," June 26, 2015, https://www.thecannabist.co/2015/06/26/photos-uruguay-marijuana-club/36742/.

70. Nick Miroff, "Inside Story on Uruguay, Where the Government Is Your Weed Dealer," *The Cannabist*, July 10, 2017, https://www.thecannabist.co/2017/07/10/uruguay-cannabis-legalization-government-sales-pharmacies/83360/.

71. Meagan Campbell, "Legalizing Weed: How Uruguay Tripped Up," *Maclean's*, March 17, 2017, http://www.macleans.ca/politics/legalizing-weed-how-uruguay-tripped-up/.

CHAPTER 6

1. Zach Sokol, "A Stoned Swan Song: Scenes from the Lost Prohibition-Era Cannabis Competition in California, Where Big Weed Is Rising and Growers Are Getting Burnt," *Playboy*, March/April 2018, 41.

2. Ian Lovett, "Where Cannabis Smells Like Big Business; New California Law on Marijuana Farming Draws Corporate Interest," *International New York Times*, April 12, 2016, http://www.questia.com/read/1P2-39510074/where-cannabis-smells-like-big-business-new-california.

3. Robin Abcarian, "California Is Poised to Become the Center of Cannabis Culture," *Los Angeles Times*, May 16, 2016, http://www.latimes.com/local/abcarian/la-me-abcarian-cannabis-book-20160516-story.html.

4. Dana Goodyear, "California Makes Marijuana a Wellness Industry," *The New Yorker*, January 31, 2018, https://www.newyorker.com/culture/photo-booth/california-makes-marijuana-a-wellness-industry?irgwc=1&source=affiliate_impactpmx_12f6tote_desktop_VigLink&mbid=affiliate_impactpmx_12f6tote_desktop_VigLink.

5. Max A. Cherney, "Marijuana Is Legal in California, but Buying It Is Neither Cheap nor Always Easy," *MarketWatch*, January 7, 2018, https://www.marketwatch.com/story/marijuana-is-legal-in-california-but-buying-it-is-neither-cheap-nor-always-easy-2018-01-04.

6. Jeremy Berke, "California's Cannabis Market Is Expected to Soar to $5.1 Billion—and It's Going to Be Bigger Than Beer," *Business Insider*, February 28, 2018, http://www.businessinsider.com/california-legalizing-weed-on-january-1-market-size-revenue-2017-12.

7. "California Reaps $60 Million in Marijuana Tax Revenue, Loses $7 Billion to Gig Economy," *420 Intel*, May 15, 2018, http://420intel.com/articles/2018/05/15/california-reaps-60-million-marijuana-tax-revenue-loses-7-billion-gig-economy?utm_source=420+Intel+-+Marijuana+Industry+News&utm_campaign=1d3fedc3cd-420+Intel&utm_medium=email&utm_term=0_3210cbef52-1d3fedc3cd-274925957.

8. Marisa Kendall, "Edibles Feast: Companies Ready to Grab a Big Piece of California's Recreational Marijuana Market," *The Cannabist*, May 30, 2017, http://www.thecannabist.co/2017/05/30/california-recreational-marijuana-sales-edibles/80392/.

9. Amanda Chicago Lewis, "Ten Popular Weed Products That Could Soon Be Illegal under Proposed Regulations," *LAist*, May 15, 2017, http://laist.com/2017/05/15/weed_products.php.

10. Joseph Misulonas, "California Edibles Makers Are Being Shut Out by the State," *Civilized*, March 27, 2018, https://www.civilized.life/articles/california-edibles-makers-shut-out/.

11. Elise McDonough, "California's Marijuana Edibles Makers Are Going Extinct," *GreenState*, March 26, 2018, http://www.greenstate.com/news/california-marijuana-edibles-makers-are-going-extinct/.

12. Elise McDonough, "California's Cannabis Edibles Just Got Surprisingly Boring," *Vice Munchies*, January 8, 2018, https://munchies.vice.com/en_us/article/3k55qj/californias-cannabis-edibles-just-got-surprisingly-boring.

13. William Sumner, "The Rise of Cannawine—Cannabis-Infused Wine," *Green Market Report*, April 4, 2018, https://www.greenmarketreport.com/the-rise-of-cannawine-cannabis-infused-wine/.

14. "Only One in Seven California Cities Allow Recreational Marijuana Stores," *420Intel*, April 16, 2018, http://420intel.com/articles/2018/04/16/only-one-seven-california-cities-allow-recreational-marijuana-stores?utm_source=420+Intel+-+Marijuana+Industry+News&utm_campaign=0e02b9ca44-420+Intel&utm_medium=email&utm_term=0_3210cbef52-0e02b9ca44-274925957.

15. Brooke Staggs, "High Marijuana Taxes Spark Sticker Shock for California Cannabis Customers," *Pasadena Star-News*, January 26, 2018, http://www.questia.com/read/1P4-1991581406/high-marijuana-taxes-spark-sticker-shock-for-california.

16. Zach Harris, "California's Legal Weed Sales Are Lagging Behind Expectations, Analysts Say," *Merry Jane*, April 11, 2018, https://merryjane.com/news/california-legal-weed-sales-lagging-behind-expectations-analysts-say.

17. Harris, "California's Legal Weed Sales."

18. Althia Raj, "Trudeau Tells Senators to Pass His Government's Marijuana Legalization Bill," *Huffington Post*, March 22, 2018, https://www.huffingtonpost.ca/2018/03/22/trudeau-senate-pot-marijuana-vote_a_23392813/.

19. Julie Weed, "Move Over California—Canada's Opening Its Own $5B Cannabis Market in 2018," *Forbes*, December 18, 2017, https://www.forbes

.com/sites/julieweed/2017/12/18/never-mind-california-canadas-opening-its-own-5b-cannabis-market-in-2018/#5e15f38a5ae6.

20. Celia Carr, "New Report from CIBC Expects Legal Cannabis Sales in Canada Will Top Alcohol Sales by 2020," *420 Intel*, May 9, 2018, http://420intel.com/articles/2018/05/09/new-report-cibc-expects-legal-cannabis-sales-canada-will-top-alcohol-sales-2020?utm_source=420%20Intel%20-%20Marijuana%20Industry%20News&utm_campaign=8feba2e2af-420%20Intel&utm_medium=email&utm_term=0_3210cbef52-8feba2e2af-274925957.

21. Oliver Bennett, "Canada's Rocky Road Journey to Legalising Cannabis," *Independent*, October 16, 2017, https://www.independent.co.uk/news/long_reads/canada-cannabis-legal-justin-trudeau-decriminalise-weed-journey-a7996696.html.

22. Patricia G. Erickson, "Recent Trends in Canadian Drug Policy: The Decline and Resurgence of Prohibitionism," *Daedalus* 121, no. 3 (Summer 1992): 239–67, 241.

23. Emily F. Murphy, *The Black Candle* (Toronto: Thomas Allen, 1922), 333, https://archive.org/details/TheBlackCandle.

24. Catherine Carstairs and University of Guelph, "How Pot-Smoking Became Illegal in Canada," *Canadian Press*, March 16, 2018, http://www.questia.com/read/1P4-2014766632/how-pot-smoking-became-illegal-in-canada.

25. Erikson, "Recent Trends in Canadian Drug Policy," 239–67, 248–49.

26. Ian Austen, "In Canada, Growing Cannabis Goes Corporate; New Rules Make Way for Large-Scale Production of Medical Marijuana," *International New York Times*, May 26, 2014, http://www.questia.com/read/1P2-38009691/in-canada-growing-cannabis-goes-corporate-new-rules.

27. Alexandra Gill, "It's High Time Vancouver Hopped on the Weed Tourism Boat," *Vv*, April 20, 2015, http://viewthevibe.com/its-high-time-vancouver-hopped-on-the-weed-tourism-boat/.

28. Danny Kruger, "How to Make Cannabis Boring," *The Spectator*, March 11, 2017, http://www.questia.com/read/1P4-1917480006/how-to-make-cannabis-boring.

29. Jacquie Miller, "Cannabis Gummy Bears and Cookies: Edible Products Pose a Challenge as Canada Moves to Legalize Pot," *Toronto Sun*, June 18, 2017, http://m.torontosun.com/2017/06/18/cannabis-gummy-bears-and-cookies-edible-products-pose-a-challenge-as-canada-moves-to-legalize-pot.

30. Jonathan Hiltz, "Can I Make Money with Cannabis Edibles?" *Food in Canada*, April 24, 2018, http://www.foodincanada.com/food-in-canada/cannabis-edibles-139546/.

31. Salma Ibrahim, "Brownies and Beer: How Edible Cannabis Businesses Plan to Cash in on Legalization," *CBC News*, February 13, 2018, http://www.cbc.ca/news/canada/toronto/joint-ventures-edibles-1.4532562.

32. "In Canada, Marijuana Edible Sales Delayed Even as Interest Among Canadians Grows," *Entrepreneur*, October 17, 2017, https://www.entrepreneur.com/article/302736?mc_cid=d70d298e7d&mc_eid=19320b5337.

33. Rebecca Harris, "The New 'Baked' Goods: Canada's New Marijuana Legislation Could Open up Big Opportunities for Makers of Edibles," *Food in Canada*, February 26, 2018, http://www.foodincanada.com/features/new-baked-goods/.

34. Scott Wilson, "Outlaw Weed Comes into the Light," *Washington Post*, March 16, 2018, https://www.washingtonpost.com/news/national/wp/2018/03/16/feature/californias-outlaw-marijuana-culture-faces-a-harsh-reckoning-legal-weed/?utm_term=.2d18a996b78b.

35. Brad Branan, "Growers Association Sues State over Large-Scale Marijuana Farms in California," *Sacramento Bee*, January 24, 2018, http://www.sacbee.com/news/state/california/california-weed/article196400149.html.

36. Mike Adams, "6 Cannabis Industry Trends Shaping the Future of Pot," *Cannabis Now*, April 16, 2018, https://cannabisnow.com/cannabis-industry-trends/.

37. Alicia Wallace, "How One of America's Most Visible Fortune 1000 Giants Quietly Snuck into the Cannabis Industry," *The Cannabist*, September 22, 2016, https://www.thecannabist.co/2016/09/22/scotts-miracle-gro-cannabis-hawthorne-gardening-co-hydroponics/61763/.

38. Alicia Wallace, "Scotts Miracle-Gro in Talks with EPA about Marijuana Pesticides," *The Cannabist*, November 4, 2016, https://www.thecannabist.co/2016/11/04/scotts-marijuana-pesticides-epa-talks/66773/.

39. Jennifer Long, "George Soros and Big Agriculture Move the Marijuana Movement," Geopolitika.ru, https://www.geopolitica.ru/en/837-george-soros-and-big-agriculture-move-the-marijuana-movement.html.

40. Dan Alexander, "Cannabis Capitalist: Scotts Miracle-Gro CEO Bets Big on Pot Growers," *Forbes*, July 26, 2016, https://www.forbes.com/sites/danalexander/2016/07/06/cannabis-capitalist-scotts-miracle-gro-ceo-bets-big-on-pot-growers/#694b80f86155.

41. "Farmers Overwhelmingly Oppose Bayer Monsanto Merger," FarmAid.org, March 8, 2018, https://www.farmaid.org/issues/corporate-power/farmers-overwhelmingly-oppose-bayer-monsanto-merger/.

42. Alex Halperin, "Chem Tales: What Will the Bayer-Monsanto Merger Mean for Cannabis?" *San Francisco Weekly,* September 28, 2016, http://www.sfweekly.com/news/chemtales/chem-tales-will-bayer-monsanto-merger-mean-cannabis/.

43. Carrie Arnold, "The Rise of Marijuana™ (Patent Pending)," *Nova Next*, October 19, 2016, http://www.pbs.org/wgbh/nova/next/evolution/patenting-pot/.

44. Amanda Chicago Lewis, "The Great Pot Monopoly Mystery," *GQ*, August 23, 2017, https://www.gq.com/story/the-great-pot-monopoly-mystery?mc_cid=c611164cc9&mc_eid=19320b5337.

45. Mike Adams, "Many Vegetable Growers Want to Transition to Marijuana," *Fresh Toast*, January 29, 2018, https://thefreshtoast.com/cannabis/many-vegetable-growers-want-transition-marijuana/.

46. Adams, "6 Cannabis Industry Trends."

47. Brent Bambury, "Big Weed: Why Legalization Isn't Necessarily a Boon for Craft Cannabis Producers," CBC Radio, May 19, 2018, http://www.cbc.ca/radio/day6/episode-390-how-conflict-helps-netanyahu-harry-and-meghan-chasing-lava-corporate-weed-deadpool-2-and-more-1.4666331/big-weed-why-legalization-isn-t-necessarily-a-boon-for-craft-cannabis-producers-1.4666338.

48. "Canopy Growth Enters 5th Continent with $29 Million African Cannabis Producer Acquisition," *New Cannabis Ventures*, May 30, 2018, https://www.newcannabisventures.com/canopy-growth-enters-5th-continent-with-29-million-african-cannabis-producer-acquisition/.

49. Sean Williams, "The Largest Pot Stock in the World Is Moving to the NYSE," May 21, 2018, https://www.fool.com/investing/2018/05/21/the-largest-pot-stock-in-the-world-is-moving-to-th.aspx.

50. "Cannabis May Be the Next Trend for a 'Desperate' Food Industry," *Lift*, December 30, 2016, https://news.lift.co/cannabis-may-be-the-next-trend-for-a-desperate-food-industry/amp/.

51. Faith Popcorn, "Investing in the Future," *Food & Drink*, September 22, 2017, http://www.fooddrink-magazine.com/sections/columns/2288-investing-in-the-future.

52. "The Marijuana Industry's Newest Spokesman? Former House Speaker John Boehner," *Fortune*, April 11, 2018, http://fortune.com/2018/04/11/pot-marijuana-john-boehner-speaker-republican/.

Bibliography

Abcarian, Robin. "California Is Poised to Become the Center of Cannabis Culture." *Los Angeles Times*, May 16, 2016. http://www.latimes.com/local/abcarian/la-me-abcarian-cannabis-book-20160516-story.html.

Abel, E. L. *Marihuana: The First Twelve Thousand Years*. New York: Springer Publishing, 1980.

Abrahamian, Atossa Araxia. "Baking Bad: A Potted History of 'High Times.'" *The Nation*, October 30, 2013. https://www.thenation.com/article/baking-bad-potted-history-high-times/.

Adams, Mike. "Many Vegetable Growers Want to Transition to Marijuana." *Fresh Toast*, January 29, 2018. https://thefreshtoast.com/cannabis/many-vegetable-growers-want-transition-marijuana/.

Adams, Mike. "6 Cannabis Industry Trends Shaping the Future of Pot." *Cannabis Now*, April 16, 2018. https://cannabisnow.com/cannabis-industry-trends/.

Alexander, Dan. "Cannabis Capitalist: Scotts Miracle-Gro CEO Bets Big on Pot Growers." *Forbes*, July 26, 2016. https://www.forbes.com/sites/danalexander/2016/07/06/cannabis-capitalist-scotts-miracle-gro-ceo-bets-big-on-pot-growers/#694b80f86155.

"Alice B. Toklas Reads Her Famous Recipe for Hashish Fudge." *Open Culture*, January 22, 2014. http://www.openculture.com/2014/01/alice-b-toklas-talks-about-her-famous-recipe-for-hashish-fudge.html.

"Alice Toklas, 89, Is Dead in Paris." *New York Times*, March 8, 1967. https://archive.nytimes.com/www.nytimes.com/books/98/05/03/specials/stein-toklasobit.html?_r=1&oref=slogin.

Andre, Christelle M., Jean-Francois Hausman, and Gea Guerriero. "*Cannabis sativa*: The Plant of the Thousand and One Molecules." *Frontiers in Plant Science* 7, no. 19 (2016).

Angus, Meagan. "Remembering the Florence Nightingale of Medical Marijuana." *Seattle Weekly*, June 29, 2016. http://www.seattleweekly.com/food/remembering-the-florence-nightingale-of-medical-marijuana/.

Anslinger, Harry Jacob. *Marijuana: Assassin of Youth.* New York: Crowell Publishing, 1937.

Arnold, Carrie. "The Rise of Marijuana™ (Patent Pending)." *Nova Next*, PBS, October 19, 2016. http://www.pbs.org/wgbh/nova/next/evolution/patenting-pot/.

Austen, Ian. "In Canada, Growing Cannabis Goes Corporate; New Rules Make Way for Large-Scale Production of Medical Marijuana." *International New York Times*, May 26, 2014. http://www.questia.com/read/1P2-38009691/in-canada-growing-cannabis-goes-corporate-new-rules.

Bachelard, Michael. "Coffee and Ganja Provide a Healthy Income in Aceh." *Sydney Morning Herald*, January 11, 2015. https://www.smh.com.au/world/coffee-and-ganja-provide-a-healthy-income-in-aceh-20150111-12ltev.html.

Baltin, Steve. "Meet the Herbal Chef, the Man Turning Weed-Infused Food Gourmet." *Forbes*, December 5, 2017. https://www.forbes.com/sites/stevebaltin/2017/12/05/meet-the-herbal-chef-the-man-turning-weed-infused-food-gourmet/#248058c5b246.

Bambury, Brent. "Big Weed: Why Legalization Isn't Necessarily a Boon for Craft Cannabis Producers." CBC Radio, May 19, 2018. http://www.cbc.ca/radio/day6/episode-390-how-conflict-helps-netanyahu-harry-and-meghan-chasing-lava-corporate-weed-deadpool-2-and-more-1.4666331/big-weed-why-legalization-isn-t-necessarily-a-boon-for-craft-cannabis-producers-1.4666338.

Barcott, Bruce. "The Great Marijuana Experiment: A Tale of Two Drug Wars." *Rolling Stone*, January 3, 2014. https://www.rollingstone.com/politics/news/the-great-marijuana-experiment-a-tale-of-two-drug-wars-20140103.

Barrett, Leonard Sr. *The Rastafarians.* Boston, MA: Beacon Press, 1997.

Barrus, D. G., K. L. Capogrossi, S. C. Cates, et al. "Tasty THC: Promises and Challenges of Cannabis Edibles." *Methods Report (RTI Press)*, November 2016. https://www.ncbi.nlm.nih.gov/pmc/articles/PMC5260817/.

Baudelaire, Charles. *Artificial Paradises: Baudelaire's Masterpiece on Hashish.* New York: Citadel, 1998.

Baudelaire, Charles. "The Poems of Hashish." Erowid.org. https://www.erowid.org/culture/characters/baudelaire_charles/baudelaire_charles_poem1.shtml.Baum, Dan. "Legalize It All." *Harper's*, April 2016. https://harpers.org/archive/2016/04/legalize-it-all/.

Bennett, Chris. "The Incredible, Delectable, Miracle of 19th Century Medicine: Hasheesh Candy!" *Cannabis Culture*, February 7, 2013. https://

www.cannabisculture.com/content/2013/02/07/incredible-delectable-miracle-19th-century-medicine-hasheesh-candy.

Bennett, Oliver. "Canada's Rocky Road Journey to Legalising Cannabis." *Independent*, October 16, 2017. https://www.independent.co.uk/news/long_reads/canada-cannabis-legal-justin-trudeau-decriminalise-weed-journey-a7996696.html.

Berke, Jeremy. "California's Cannabis Market Is Expected to Soar to $5.1 Billion—and It's Going to Be Bigger Than Beer." *Business Insider*, February 28, 2018. http://www.businessinsider.com/california-legalizing-weed-on-january-1-market-size-revenue-2017-12.

Bienenstock, David. "7 Cannabis Edibles That Changed the Game." *Leafly*, February 22, 2018. https://www.leafly.com/news/strains-products/7-weed-edibles-that-changed-the-game.

Birdsall, John. "Jeremiah Tower's Invincible Armor of Pleasure." *Eater*, November 7, 2014. https://www.eater.com/2014/11/7/7166097/jeremiah-towers-invincible-armor-of-pleasure.

Blackman, Shane. *Chilling Out: The Cultural Politics of Substance Consumption, Youth and Drug Policy*. Maidenhead, England: Open University Press, 2003.

Bradshaw, Jon. "The Reggae Way to 'Salvation.'" *New York Times*, August 14, 1977.

Branan, Brad. "Growers Association Sues State over Large-Scale Marijuana Farms in California." *Sacramento Bee*, January 24, 2018. http://www.sacbee.com/news/state/california/california-weed/article196400149.html.

Bruner, Belinda. "A Recipe for Modernism and the Somatic Intellect in the *Alice B. Toklas Cook Book* and Gertrude Stein's 'Tender Buttons.'" *Papers on Language & Literature* 45, no. 4 (2009): 411.

Bryant, Jackie. "San Diego Pop-Up Dinners Pair Cannabis with Food." *Eater San Diego*, February 14, 2018. https://sandiego.eater.com/2018/2/14/17011216/san-diego-cannabis-marijuana-dinners.

Burke, J. F. "Eat It!" *High Times*, February 1978, 47–49.

"California Reaps $60 Million in Marijuana Tax Revenue, Loses $7 Billion to Gig Economy." *420 Intel*, May 15, 2018. http://420intel.com/articles/2018/05/15/california-reaps-60-million-marijuana-tax-revenue-loses-7-billion-gig-economy?utm_source=420+Intel+-+Marijuana+Industry+News&utm_campaign=1d3fedc3cd-420+Intel&utm_medium=email&utm_term=0_3210cbef52-1d3fedc3cd-274925957.

Campbell, Meagan. "Legalizing Weed: How Uruguay Tripped Up." *Maclean's*, March 17, 2017. http://www.macleans.ca/politics/legalizing-weed-how-uruguay-tripped-up/.

Campos, Isaac. *Home Grown: Marijuana and the Origins of Mexico's War on Drugs*. Chapel Hill, NC: University of North Carolina Press, 2012.

Canby, Vincent. "Screen: 'I Love You, Alice B. Toklas!'" *New York Times*, October 8, 1968. https://timesmachine.nytimes.com/timesmachine/1968/10/08/76888012.pdf.

"Cannabis May Be the Next Trend for a 'Desperate' Food Industry." *Lift*, December 30, 2016. https://news.lift.co/cannabis-may-be-the-next-trend for-a-desperate-food-industry/amp/.

"Canopy Growth Enters 5th Continent with $29 Million African Cannabis Producer Acquisition." *New Cannabis Ventures*, May 30, 2018. https://www.newcannabisventures.com/canopy-growth-enters-5th-continent-with-29-million-african-cannabis-producer-acquisition/.

Carr, Celia. "New Report from CIBC Expects Legal Cannabis Sales in Canada Will Top Alcohol Sales by 2020." *420 Intel*, May 9, 2018. http://420intel.com/articles/2018/05/09/new-report-cibc-expects-legal-cannabis-sales-canada-will-top-alcohol-sales-2020?utm_source=420%20Intel%20-%20Marijuana%20Industry%20News&utm_campaign=8feba2e2af-420%20Intel&utm_medium=email&utm_term=0_3210cbef52-8feba2e2af-274925957.

Carstairs, Catherine, and University of Guelph. "How Pot-Smoking Became Illegal in Canada." *Canadian Press*, March 16, 2018. http://www.questia.com/read/1P4-2014766632/how-pot-smoking-became-illegal-in-canada.

Cervantes, Jorges. "The Reign of Spain: A Festive Mediterranean Lifestyle and Favorable Laws Have Made Spain the New Cannabis Capital of Europe." *High Times*, June 2004, 31.

Cherney, Max A. "Marijuana Is Legal in California, but Buying It Is Neither Cheap nor Always Easy." *MarketWatch*, January 7, 2018. https://www.marketwatch.com/story/marijuana-is-legal-in-california-but-buying-it-is-neither-cheap-nor-always-easy-2018-01-04.

Clarke, Robert C., and Mark D. Merlin. *Cannabis: Evolution and Ethnobotany*. Berkeley, CA: University of California Press, 2013.

Clarke, Robert C., and Mark D. Merlin. "Cannabis Taxonomy: The 'Sativa' vs. 'Indica' Debate." *HerbalGram*, 2016.

"Code of Conduct for European Cannabis Social Clubs," December 9, 2011. http://www.encod.org/info/CODE-OF-CONDUCT-FOR-EUROPEAN.html.

"Coffee Shops in Amsterdam: Why Are the Amsterdam Cannabis Cafes Allowed?" http://www.amsterdam-advisor.com/coffee-shops-in-amsterdam.html.

Cohen, Ira. "The Goblet of Dreams." *Playboy*, April 1966, 125–28.

"Colorado Cannabis and the Use of Pesticides: Where Are We At?" *The Cannabist*, May 19, 2016. https://www.thecannabist.co/2016/05/19/colorado-cannabis-pesticides-update/54430/.

Connerney, Richard. *The Upside-Down Tree: India's Changing Culture.* New York: Algora, 2009.

"Cops Pop 'Brownie Mary.'" *High Times*, May 1981, 2.

Courtney, William. "Cannabis as a Unique Functional Food." *Treating Yourself* 24 (2010): 54.

Danko, Danny. "Spain." *High Times*, December 2013, 50.

Davidson, Alan. *The Oxford Companion to Food.* Oxford, UK: Oxford University Press, 2014.

Davis, Stephen. "Fear in Paradise." *New York Times*, July 25, 1976, 153.

Deitch, Robert. *Hemp: American History Revisited—the Plant with a Divided History.* New York: Algora, 2003.

Donohue, Caitlin. "La Abuela: Fernanda de la Figuera Is Spain's Grandmother of Marijuana." *SF Evergreen*, May 20, 2015. http://sfevergreen.com/la-abuela-fernanda-de-la-figuera-is-spains-grandmother-of-marijuana/.

Dowd, Maureen. "Don't Harsh Our Mellow, Dude." *New York Times*, June 3, 2014. https://www.nytimes.com/2014/06/04/opinion/dowd-dont-harsh-our-mellow-dude.html.

"Drive on Narcotics Sped by Treasury; Campaign to Rid the Nation of Marijuana Is a Feature of Year's Program." *New York Times*, January 31, 1938, 12.

Duchess of York Sarah. "The Battle for Medical Marijuana." *The Nation*, January 6, 1997. http://www.questia.com/read/1G1-18994067/the-battle-for-medical-marijuana.

Dumas, Alexandre. *The Count of Monte Cristo.* London: Chapman and Hall, 1844.

Earlywine, Mitch. *Understanding Marijuana: A New Look at the Scientific Evidence.* Oxford, England, UK: Oxford University Press, 2005.

Ebert, Roger. "I Love You, Alice B. Toklas." November 27, 1968. https://www.rogerebert.com/reviews/i-love-you-alice-b-toklas-1968.

Ebert, Roger. *The Great Movies IV.* Chicago: University of Chicago Press, 2016.

Elwin, Verrier. "The Origin of Ganja." In *Wildest Dreams: An Anthology of Drug-Related Literature*, edited by Richard Rudgley, 96–97. London: Thistle Publishing, 2014.

Emerson Sen, Gertrude. *Voiceless India*, revised edition. New York: John Day Company, 1944.

Eplett, Layla. "Go Ask Alice: The History of Toklas' Legendary Hashish Fudge." *Scientific American*, April 20, 2015. https://blogs.scientificamerican.com/food-matters/go-ask-alice-the-history-of-toklas-8217-legendary-hashish-fudge/.

Erickson, Patricia G. "Recent Trends in Canadian Drug Policy: The Decline and Resurgence of Prohibitionism." *Daedalus* 121, no. 3 (Summer 1992): 239–67.

Eriksen, Lars Hinnerskov. "Cooking with Cannabis—a New Culinary High?" *The Guardian*, January 7, 2014. https://www.theguardian.com/lifeandstyle/wordofmouth/2014/jan/07/cooking-cannabis-culinary-high-novelty-ingredient-hemp-chefs.

Erkelens, Jacob L., and Arno Hazekamp. "That Which We Call *Indica*, by Any Other Name Would Smell as Sweet." *Cannabinoids 2014*.

"Farmers Overwhelmingly Oppose Bayer Monsanto Merger." FarmAid.org, March 8, 2018. https://www.farmaid.org/issues/corporate-power/farmers-overwhelmingly-oppose-bayer-monsanto-merger/.

Farrell, Barry. "The Other Culture: An Explorer of the Worldwide Underground of Art Finds, Behind Its Orgiastic Happenings, Brutalities and Pot-Seed Pancakes, a Wild Utopian Dream." *Life*, February 17, 1967, 87–94.

Flaccus, Gillian. "Marijuana Growers Turning to Hemp as CBD Extract Explodes." AP News, May 14, 2018. https://www.apnews.com/9d36d2784bf94c7684f03b014989e17f/Marijuana-growers-turning-to-hemp-as-CBD-extract-explodes.

Flatt, Courtney. "Can the Cannabis Industry Deliver an Organic, Environmentally Sensitive High?" OPB.org, December 23, 2016. https://www.opb.org/news/article/organically-grown-marijuana/.

Fort, Joel. "Pot: A Rational Approach." *Playboy*, October 1, 1969, 130.

Frater, Adrian. "No to Edible Ganja Products—Ras Iyah V . . . Calls for Cannabis-Oriented Educational Programmes." *Jamaica Gleaner*, May 31, 2017. http://jamaica-gleaner.com/article/lead-stories/20170531/no-edible-ganja-products-ras-iyah-v-calls-cannabis-oriented.

Gagliardi, Marcia. "Underground Cannabis Dinners Are Creating Quite a Buzz in the Bay Area (and Wine Is No Longer the Primary Food Pairing)." KQED.org, December 29, 2017. https://www.kqed.org/bayareabites/124226/underground-cannabis-dinners-are-creating-quite-a-buzz-in-the-bay-area-and-wine-is-no-longer-the-primary-food-pairing.

Garner, Dwight. "Trusting in *The Sheltering Sky*, Even When It Scorched." *New York Times*, August 30, 2009. https://www.nytimes.com/2009/08/31/books/31bowles.html.

Geerlings, P. J. "Treatment of Drug Addicts." *Maandblad voor Geestelijke Volksgezondheid* 30, no. 11 (1975): 4952.

Geiger, John. *Nothing Is True, Everything Is Permitted: The Life of Brion Gysin*. New York: Disinformation Books, 2005.

Gianakos, Mike. "500 Issues of *High Times*: A History of the World's Most Notorious Magazine." HighTimes.com, August 30, 2017. https://hightimes.com/culture/500-issues-of-high-times-a-history-of-the-worlds-most-notorious-magazine/.

Gieringer, Dale. "A Warning Re Dabs." *O'Shaughnessy's* Online. http://www beyondthc.com/a-warning-re-dabs/.

Gill, Alexandra. "It's High Time Vancouver Hopped on the Weed Tourism Boat." *Vv*, April 20, 2015. http://viewthevibe.com/its-high-time-vancouver-hopped-on-the-weed-tourism-boat/.

Gillespie, Nick. "Prescription: Drugs." *Reason*, February 1997. http://www.questia.com/read/1G1-19192456/prescription-drugs.

Gliha, Lori Jane, and Serene Fang. "Colorado Cannabis Czar: We Didn't Anticipate Problems with Pot Edibles." *Al Jazeera*, January 7, 2015. http://america.aljazeera.com/watch/shows/america-tonight/articles/2015/1/7/colorado-cannabisczarwedidntanticipateproblemswithpotedibles.html.

Goldberg, Carey. "Marijuana Club Helps Those in Pain." *The New York Times*, February 25, 1996. https://www.nytimes.com/1996/02/25/us/marijuana-club-helps-those-in-pain.html.

Goldberg, Carey. "Brownie Mary Fights to Legalize Marijuana." *New York Times*, July 6, 1996. https://www.nytimes.com/1996/07/06/us/brownie-mary-fights-to-legalize-marijuana.html.

Goldfield, Hannah. "A Marijuana Dinner Party Grows Underground." *The New Yorker*, March 8, 2018. https://www.newyorker.com/culture/tables-for-two/an-underground-marijuana-dinner-party-grows-in-new-york?mbid=social_facebook.

Goni, Uki. "High Times in Montevideo: Uruguay Entering Brave New World of Pot Legalization." *Time*, August 5, 2013. http://world.time.com/2013/08/05/high-times-in-montevideo-uruguay-enters-brave-new-world-of-pot-legalization/.

Goode, Erich, ed. *Marijuana*. Chicago: Atherton, 1969.

Goodyear, Dana. "California Makes Marijuana a Wellness Industry." *The New Yorker*, January 31, 2018. https://www.newyorker.com/culture/photo-booth/california-makes-marijuana-a-wellness-industry?irgwc=1&source=affiliate_impactpmx_12f6tote_desktop_VigLink&mbid=affiliate_impactpmx_12f6tote_desktop_VigLink.

Gorman, Peter. "Indonesia: Smokin' on Sumatra." *High Times*, September 1984, 49.

Gorman, Peter. "Brownie Mary Busted: Faces Five Years for Baking Magic Brownies for PWAs." *High Times*, December 1992, 23.

Gorman, Peter. "Interview: Brownie Mary Rathburn." *High Times*, January 1993, 50–59.

Gorman, Peter. "Cambodia: Where Marijuana Is Legal." *High Times*, September 1994, 49.

Gorman, Peter. "Feds Fly Anti-Pot Doc Balloon." *High Times*, April 1997, 20.

Grimm, Beca. "Baked to Perfection: This Stoned Scone Goes Perfectly with Your 'Tea' HC." *Merry Jane*, August 9, 2017. https://merryjane.com/culture/baked-to-perfection-jessica-coles-date-scones-white-rabbit-high-tea.

Grinspoon, Lester. *Marihuana Reconsidered.* Cambridge, MA: Harvard University Press, 1971.

Grinspoon, Lester. "Opium, not Alcohol, Is the Demon." *New York Times*, October 24, 1971.

Grinspoon, Lester. "Cannabis Clubs: Public Nuisance or Therapy?" *Playboy*, November 1998, 44.

Gstalter, Morgan. "McConnell Bill Would Legalize Hemp as Agricultural Product." *The Hill*, March 26, 2018. http://thehill.com/policy/energy-environment/380287-mcconnell-bill-would-legalize-hemp-as-agricultural-product.

Gunelius, Susan. "Is Hemp the Biggest Opportunity in the Cannabis Market?" *Cannabiz*, February 20, 2018. https://cannabiz.media/hemp-opportunity-cannabis-market/.

Haberkorn, Leonardo. "'Gourmet Cannabis': Take a Peek Inside a Uruguay Marijuana Club." June 26, 2015. https://www.thecannabist.co/2015/06/26/photos-uruguay-marijuana-club/36742/.

Haberman, David L. *Journey through the Twelve Forests: An Encounter with Krishna.* New York: Oxford University Press, 1994.

Hacker, Daphna. "Colonialism's Civilizing Mission: The Case of the Indian Hemp Drugs Commission." Tel Aviv University, 2001, 458. http://law.bepress.com/cgi/viewcontent.cgi?article=1161&context=taulwps.

Haines, Gavin. "Why Amsterdam's Oldest Cannabis 'Coffeeshop' Has Been Forced to Close." *Telegraph*, January 3, 2017. https://www.telegraph.co.uk/travel/destinations/europe/netherlands/amsterdam/articles/amsterdams-oldest-coffeeshop-mellow-yellow-is-forced-to-close/

Halperin, Alex. "Chem Tales: What Will the Bayer-Monsanto Merger Mean for Cannabis?" *San Francisco Weekly*, September 28, 2016. http://www.sfweekly.com/news/chemtales/chem-tales-will-bayer-monsanto-merger-mean-cannabis/.

Harfenist, Ethan, and Bennett Murray. "The High Life." *Phnom Penh Post*, May 29, 2015. https://www.phnompenhpost.com/post-weekend/high-life.

Harris, Rebecca. "The New 'Baked' Goods: Canada's New Marijuana Legislation Could Open Up Big Opportunities for Makers of Edibles." *Food in Canada*, February 26, 2018. http://www.foodincanada.com/features/new-baked-goods/.

Harris, Zach. "California's Legal Weed Sales Are Lagging Behind Expectations, Analysts Say." *Merry Jane*, April 11, 2018. https://merryjane.com/news/california-legal-weed-sales-lagging-behind-expectations-analysts-say.

Healy, Jack. "New Scrutiny on Sweets with Ascent of Marijuana in Colorado." *New York Times*, October 29, 2014. https://www.nytimes.com/2014/10/30/us/new-scrutiny-on-sweets-with-ascent-of-marijuana-in-colorado.html.

Hecht, Peter. *Weed Land: Inside America's Marijuana Epicenter and How Pot Went Legit.* Oakland: University of California Press, 2014.

Henninger, Danya. "David Ansill's Next Act: Marijuana-Infused Pop-Up Dinners." *Billypenn*, January 29, 2017. https://billypenn.com/2017/01/29/david-ansills-next-act-marijuana-infused-pop-up-dinners/.

Herer, Jack. *The Emperor Wears No Clothes: Hemp and the Marijuana Conspiracy.* Van Nuys, CA: Ah Ha Publishing, 1985.

Hiltz, Jonathan. "Can I Make Money with Cannabis Edibles?" *Food in Canada*, April 24, 2018. http://www.foodincanada.com/food-in-canada/cannabis-edibles-139546/.

Hirsch, Jesse. "Local Cannabis Chefs Are Out to Prove Their Dinners Can Be More Than Dope." *Edible Brooklyn*, March 23, 2017. https://www.ediblebrooklyn.com/2017/local-cannabis-chefs-prove-dinners-more-dope/.

Hoch, Jeanna. "Stories of Amendment 64 Oral History Project." Jeanna Hoch, interviewed by Janet Bishop (Colorado State Library). https://dspace.library.colostate.edu/handle/10217/176470.

Hodgson, Moira. "Review: The American 'Gourmands' Way' through France." *Wall Street Journal*, November 17, 2017. https://www.wsj.com/articles/review-the-american-gourmands-way-through-france-1510955459.

Hong, Shao, and Robert C. Clarke. "1996 Taxonomic Studies of Cannabis in China." http://www.hempfood.com/iha/iha03207.html.

"Hooray! The Bulldog Turned 40 in 2015!" https://www.thebulldog.com/40-years-the-living-room-of-amsterdam/.

Hutchcraft, Jak. "The Roots of Cannabis Slang." Prohbtd.com, October 22, 2017. https://prohbtd.com/the-roots-of-cannabis-slang.

Ibrahim, Salma. "Brownies and Beer: How Edible Cannabis Businesses Plan to Cash in on Legalization." *CBC News*, February 13, 2018. http://www.cbc.ca/news/canada/toronto/joint-ventures-edibles-1.4532562.

"I Love You, Alice B. Toklas!" *Variety*, December 31, 1967. http://variety.com/1967/film/reviews/i-love-you-alice-b-toklas-1200421625/.

"In Canada, Marijuana Edible Sales Delayed Even as Interest among Canadians Grows." *Entrepreneur*, October 17, 2017. https://www.entrepreneur.com/article/302736?mc_cid=d70d298e7d&mc_eid=19320b5337.

James, Wanda. "Stories of Amendment 64 Oral History Project." Wanda James, interviewed by Janet Bishop (Colorado State Library). https://dspace.library.colostate.edu/bitstream/handle/10217/176473/AMNT_OralHistoryTranscript_James-part1-sect1.pdf?sequence=1&isAllowed=y.

Jansen, A. C. M. "The Economics of Cannabis-Cultivation in Europe." Paper presented at the Second European Conference on Drug Trafficking and Law Enforcement. Paris, September 26 and 27, 2002. http://www.cedro-uva.org/lib/jansen.economics.html.

Jenison, David. "Just How Racist Was *Reefer Madness*." Prohbtd.com. https://prohbtd.com/just-how-racist-was-reefer-madness.

Jenison, David. "Meet the Duo Behind NYC's Hottest Cannabis Speakeasies." Prohibtd.com. https://prohbtd.com/meet-the-duo-behind-nycs-hottest-cannabis-speakeasies.

Kane, H. H. "A Hashish House in New York." *Harper's* 667, November 1883, 944–49.

Kaskey, Jack. "Pot Laced with Pesticides Forces States to Act as EPA Stays Away." *Bloomberg*, August 2, 2017. https://www.bloomberg.com/news/articles/2017-08-02/pot-laced-with-pesticides-forces-states-to-act-as-epa-stays-away.

Kemper, Benjamin. "The Quest for an Ancient Culture's Cannabis-Filled Cooking." *Atlas Obscura*, May 2, 2018. https://www.atlasobscura.com/articles/cannabis-cooking-in-georgia?utm_source=Gastro+Obscura+Weekly+E-mail&utm_campaign=2f03b5df80-EMAIL_CAMPAIGN_2018_05_07&utm_medium=email&utm_term=0_2418498528-2f03b5df80-68458689&mc_cid=2f03b5df80&mc_eid=b6753bc786.

Kendall, Marisa. "Edibles Feast: Companies Ready to Grab a Big Piece of California's Recreational Marijuana Market." *The Cannabist*, May 30, 2017. http://www.thecannabist.co/2017/05/30/california-recreational-marijuana-sales-edibles/80392/

King, Patricia, and Marc Peyser. "Pot Shots in the War on Drugs: 'Doonesbury' Mixes It Up over Marijuana." *Newsweek*, October 14, 1996, 52.

Klare, Joe. "Legal Pot's Pesticide Problem: What Can Be Done About It." *Marijuana Times*, March 24, 2017. https://www.marijuanatimes.org/legal-pots-pesticide-problem-what-can-be-done-about-it/.

Krebs, Albin, and Robert M. C. G. Thomas. "Notes on People; Alice B. Toklas Goodies." *New York Times*, Saturday, January 17, 1981. https://www.nytimes.com/1981/01/17/nyregion/notes-on-people-alice-b-toklas-goodies.html.

Kruger, Danny. "How to Make Cannabis Boring." *The Spectator*, March 11, 2017. http://www.questia.com/read/1P4-1917480006/how-to-make-cannabis-boring.

Labonne, Valerie. "The Booming Business of Cannabis in Spain." *France 24*, April 29, 2017. http://www.france24.com/en/20170428-reporters-spain-cannabis-clubs-marijuana-tourism-business-economy-illegal-production.

Laursen, Lucas. "Botany: The Cultivation of Weed." *Nature*, September 23, 2015. https://www.nature.com/articles/525S4a.

Lawrence, Robyn Griggs. "Is Cannabis Chocolate the Ultimate Edible?" *High Times*, February 13, 2017. https://hightimes.com/edibles/is-cannabis-chocolate-the-ultimate-edible/.

Lawrence, Robyn Griggs. "Terpene and Turn On!" *Sensi*, January 29, 2018. http://www.sensimag.com/2018/01/29/165814/terpene-and-turn-on.

Lawrence, Robyn Griggs. "Just Add Water." *Sensi*, Boulder/Denver edition, February 2018, 84–88.

Leary, Timothy. "Majoon and the Mind." *Playboy*, July 1966, 16.

Lewis, Amanda Chicago. "Ten Popular Weed Products That Could Soon Be Illegal under Proposed Regulations." *LAist*, May 15, 2017. http://laist.com/2017/05/15/weed_products.php.

Lewis, Amanda Chicago. "The Great Pot Monopoly Mystery." *GQ*, August 23, 2017. https://www.gq.com/story/the-great-pot-monopoly-mystery?mc_cid=c611164cc9&mc_eid=19320b5337.

Littlebury, Isaac. *The History of Herodotus, 1737*. London: Kessinger Publishing, 2010.

Lloyd, Pamela. "1974: A Century of Reefer Action in Five Years; or, Time Flies When You're Having Fun." *High Times*, 56.

Long, Jennifer. "George Soros and Big Agriculture Move the Marijuana Movement." Geopolitika.ru. https://www.geopolitica.ru/en/837-george-soros-and-big-agriculture-move-the-marijuana-movement.html.

Lovett, Ian. "Where Cannabis Smells Like Big Business; New California Law on Marijuana Farming Draws Corporate Interest." *International New York Times*, April 12, 2016. http://www.questia.com/read/1P2-39510074/where-cannabis-smells-like-big-business-new-california.

"'Low-Risk' Drug Sales Considered Acceptable: In Amsterdam, Cannabis Is High on Coffee Shop Menu." *Los Angeles Times*, November 2, 1986. http://articles.latimes.com/1986-11-02/news/mn-15818_1_coffee-shop.

Ludlow, Fitz Hugh. *The Hasheesh Eater: Being Passages from the Life of a Pythagorean*. Calgary, Alberta: Theophania Publishing, 2011.

MacCoun, Robert J. "What Can We Learn from the Dutch Cannabis Coffeeshop System?" Goldman School of Public Policy and UC Berkeley School of Law, University of California, Berkeley, CA, October 22, 2010. http://gspp.berkeley.edu/assets/uploads/research/pdf/MacCoun2011_DutchCannabisCoffeeshopSystem.pdf.

MacCoun, Robert J., and Michelle M. Mello. "Half-Baked—The Retail Promotion of Marijuana Edibles." *New England Journal of Medicine*, March 12, 2015. https://www.nejm.org/doi/full/10.1056/NEJMp1416014.

MacCoun, Robert J., and Peter Reuter. *Drug War Heresies: Learning from Other Vices, Times, and Places*. Cambridge, England: Cambridge University Press, 2001.

Mail Order Drug Paraphernalia Control Act, Hearing Before the Subcommittee on Crime of the Committee on the Judiciary, House of Representatives, Ninety-Ninth Congress, Second Session on H.R. 1625, May 8, 1986. ReInk Books, 2017.

Margolin, Madison. "Weed's Legal in Uruguay, But It Looks Nothing Like Colorado." *Jane Street*, July 11, 2017. https://janest.com/article/2017/07/11/weeds-legal-uruguay-looks-nothing-like-colorado/.

"Marijuana: Millions of Turned-On Users." *Life*, July 7, 1967, 21.

"The Marijuana Industry's Newest Spokesman? Former House Speaker John Boehner." *Fortune*, April 11, 2018. http://fortune.com/2018/04/11/pot-marijuana-john-boehner-speaker-republican/.

McDonough, Elise. *The Official High Times Cannabis Cookbook: More Than 50 Irresistible Recipes That Will Get You High.* San Francisco: Chronicle Books, 2012.

McDonough, Elise. "The *High Times* Interview: Action Bronson." *High Times*, July 2016, 104–9.

McDonough, Elise. "California's Cannabis Edibles Just Got Surprisingly Boring." *Vice Munchies*, January 8, 2018. https://munchies.vice.com/en_us/article/3k55qj/californias-cannabis-edibles-just-got-surprisingly-boring.

McDonough, Elise. "California's Marijuana Edibles Makers Are Going Extinct." *GreenState*, March 26, 2018. http://www.greenstate.com/news/california-marijuana-edibles-makers-are-going-extinct/.

McGroarty, Beth. "2015 Trends Report." *Spafinder Wellness 365*, 2015.

McPartland, John. "Cannabinoids Involved in Language Acquisition." *O'Shaughnessy's*, Summer 2009.

"McPartland's Correct(ed) Vernacular Nomenclature." *O'Shaughnessy's Online*, January 4, 2015.

McVey, Eli. "Chart: U.S. Hemp Production Soars in 2017." *Marijuana Business Daily*, March 26, 2018. https://mjbizdaily.com/chart-us-hemp-production-soars-2017/.

Mechoulam, Raphael. *Cannabinoids as Therapeutics.* New York: Springer Science & Business Media, 2006.

Meehan, Maureen. "Has Spain Become Europe's Marijuana Garden? Experts Say Si." *High Times*, June 20, 2017. https://hightimes.com/news/has-spain-become-europes-marijuana-garden-experts-say-si/.

Mikuriya, Tod. "Introduction to the Indian Hemp Drugs Commission Report." Comitas Institute for Anthropological Study. http://cifas.us/analyses/Mikuriya1.html.

Miller, Jacquie. "Cannabis Gummy Bears and Cookies: Edible Products Pose a Challenge as Canada Moves to Legalize Pot." *Toronto Sun*, June 18, 2017. http://m.torontosun.com/2017/06/18/cannabis-gummy-bears-and-cookies-edible-products-pose-a-challenge-as-canada-moves-to-legalize-pot.

Miller, Joshua. "Colorado Serves Edible Marijuana with a Side of Controversy." *Boston Globe*, September 16, 2016. https://www.hfcm.org/CMS/Images/Boston%20Globe.Colorado%20serves%20edible%20marijuana%20with%20a%20side%20of%20controversy.9.16.16.pdf.

Miroff, Nick. "Inside Story on Uruguay, Where the Government Is Your Weed Dealer." *The Cannabist*, July 10, 2017. https://www.thecannabist.co/2017/07/10/uruguay-cannabis-legalization-government-sales-pharmacies/83360/.

Misulonas, Joseph. "California Edibles Makers Are Being Shut Out by the State." *Civilized*, March 27, 2018. https://www.civilized.life/articles/california-edibles-makers-shut-out/.

Murdocco, Mariela. "Uruguay: The World's Laboratory for Marijuana Legalisation." *The Guardian*, October 4, 2013. https://www.theguardian.com/commentisfree/2013/oct/04/uruguay-legalize-marijuana-george-soros.

Murphy, Emily F. *The Black Candle.* Toronto: Thomas Allen, 1922.

Murrieta, Ed. "America's Top 10 Cannabis Chefs." *GreenState*, November 22, 2017. http://www.greenstate.com/food-travel/americas-top-10-cannabis-chefs/.

Nelson, George. "Georgia Eases Draconian Law on Cannabis Use." *The Guardian*, January 24, 2017. https://www.theguardian.com/world/2017/jan/24/georgia-eases-draconian-law-cannabis-landmark-ruling.

Netherlands Institute of Ecology. "The World's Most Spoken Language Is . . . Terpene." 2017. https://nioo.knaw.nl/en/press/worlds-most-spoken-language-isterpene.

Nimn, Sudough. "Khmer Green: The Happy Herb." *High Times*, September 1999, 65.

O'Brien, Glenn, and Gary Stimeling. "Interview: Vera Rubin." *High Times*, June 1978, 33–38.

Oliveira, Ricardo. "The Promises and Challenges of Cannabis Edibles." *Lift*, February 6, 2017. https://news.lift.co/promises-challenges-cannabis-edibles/.

O'Neil, Paul. "The Only Rebellion Around, But the Shabby Beats Bungle the Job in Arguing, Sulking and Bad Poetry." *Life*, November 30, 1959, 115–21.

"Only One in Seven California Cities Allow Recreational Marijuana Stores." *420 Intel*, April 16, 2018. http://420intel.com/articles/2018/04/16/only-one-seven-california-cities-allow-recreational-marijuana-stores?utm_source=420+Intel+-+Marijuana+Industry+News&utm_campaign=0e02b9ca44-420+Intel&utm_medium=email&utm_term=0_3210cbef52-0e02b9ca44-274925957.

Pacher, Pal, Sandor Batkai, and George Kunos. "The Endocannabinoid System as an Emerging Target of Pharmacotheraphy." *Pharmacological Reviews* 58, no. 3 (2006).

Page, Christina Orlovsky. "Cannabis Dinners Are Becoming 'Almost Socially Acceptable.'" *San Diego Magazine*, August 1, 2017. http://www.sandiegomagazine.com/San-Diego-Magazine/August-2017/Cannabis-Dinners-are-Becoming-Almost-Socially-Acceptable/.

Pampuro, Amanda. "Talk About Pot Luck! Ganja Gourmet Gets Ready for Its Next Course." *Westword*, April 19, 2017. http://www.westword.com/marijuana/ganja-gourmet-prepares-for-the-next-step-in-the-edible-evolution-8985358.

Pearson, Jesse. "Weed and Stoner Food, Together at Last." *GQ*, July 2, 2012. http://www.gq.com/story/weed-and-stoner-food-recipes-robertas-brooklyn.

Pliny. *Natural History, Books XXIV–XXVII. Vol. 7.* Cambridge, MA: Harvard University Press, 1980.

Polachek, Jen. "Getting Buzzed: Cooking with Pot." *Huffington Post*, December 6, 2017. https://www.huffingtonpost.com/saveur/cooking-with-pot_b_927648.html.

Politzer, Malia. "Barcelona's Pot Boom and Bust: The Uncertain Fate of Cannabis Clubs in 'The Amsterdam of Southern Europe.'" *Reason*, March 2016. http://www.questia.com/read/1G1-443399249/barcelona-s-pot-boom-and-bust-the-uncertain-fate.

Pollan, Michael. "How Pot Has Grown." *New York Times Magazine*, February 18, 1995. https://www.nytimes.com/1995/02/19/magazine/how-pot-has-grown.html.

Pollan, Michael. "Living with Medical Marijuana." *New York Times*, July 28, 1997. https://www.nytimes.com/1997/07/20/magazine/living-with-medical-marijuana.html.

Popcorn, Faith. "Investing in the Future." *Food & Drink*, September 22, 2017. http://www.fooddrink-magazine.com/sections/columns/2288-investing-in-the-future.

Potterton, Reg. "Amsterdam . . . " *Playboy*, March 1971, 135–39.

Putri, Dania, and Tom Blickman. "Cannabis in Indonesia: Patterns in Consumption, Production, and Policies." Transnational Institute, January 2016. https://www.tni.org/filtion-downloads/dpb_44_13012016_map_web.pdfes/publica.

Ra, Chef. "That First Joint." *High Times*, November 2007, 20.

Raj, Althia. "Trudeau Tells Senators to Pass His Government's Marijuana Legalization Bill." *Huffington Post*, March 22, 2018. https://www.huffingtonpost.ca/2018/03/22/trudeau-senate-pot-marijuana-vote_a_23392813/.

Ras Iyah V. "The Rasta Lifestyle, Ital Food, Ganja Farming in Jamaica, Ganja as Sacrament." Filmed February 2015, YouTube video, 11:08. Posted June 2017. https://www.youtube.com/watch?v=FI1tmqhOHwE.

Rätsch, Christian. *Marijuana Medicine: A World Tour of the Healing and Visionary Powers of Cannabis.* Rochester, VT: Healing Arts Press, 2001.

Rätsch, Christian, and Claudia Muller-Ebeling. *Pagan Christmas: The Plants, Spirits, and Rituals at the Origins of Yuletide.* New York: Inner Traditions, 2006.

Reed, Christopher. "'Brownie Mary' Rathbun." *The Guardian*, May 19, 1999. https://www.theguardian.com/news/1999/may/20/guardianobituaries1.

"Report of the Indian Hemp Drugs Commission, 1893–94." https://digital.nls.uk/indiapapers/browse/archive/74464868.

Robbins, Trina. "Brownie Mary: Good-Bye to a Saint." *High Times*, August 1, 1999, 22.

Rose, Panama. *The Hashish Cookbook*. Gnaoua Press, 1966.

Rose, Richard. "It's Nigh Time to Grandfather Hemp." Hemp.com, May 31, 2018. http://www.hemp.com/2018/05/its-nigh-time-to-grandfather-hemp/.

Rubin, Vera (ed.) *Cannabis and Culture*. The Hague: Mouton Publishers, 1975.

Rubin, Vera D., and Lambros Comitas. *Ganja in Jamaica: A Medical Anthropological Study of Chronic Marihuana Use*. The Hague: Moutaon De Gruyter, 1975.

Rudgley, Richard. *The Encyclopedia of Psychoactive Substances*. New York: St. Martin's Griffin, 2000.

Rudgley, Richard. "11: Psychoactive Plants." In *The Cultural History of Plants*, edited by Ghillean Prance and Mark Nesbitt. New York: Routledge, 2005.

Russo, Ethan B. "Cognoscenti of Cannabis I: Jacques-Joseph Moreau (1804–1884)." *Journal of Cannabis Therapeutics* 1 (2001). https://www.cannabis-med.org/data/pdf/2001-01-6.pdf.

Russo, Ethan B. "Clinical Endocannabinoid Deficiency (CECD): Can This Concept Explain Therapeutic Benefits of Cannabis in Migraine, Fibromyalgia, Irritable Bowel Syndrome and Other Treatment-Resistant Conditions?" *Neuro Endocrinology Letters*, 2008, 192–200.

Russo, Ethan B. "Taming THC: Potential Cannabis Synergy and Phytocannabinoid-Terpenoid Entourage Effects." *British Journal of Pharmacology*, August 2011, 1344–64.

Russo, Ethan B., and Franjo Grotenhermen. *The Handbook of Cannabis Therapeutics: From Bench to Bedside*. Binghamton, NY: The Haworth Press, 2006.

Russo, Ethan B., Hong-En Jiang, Xiao Li, Alan Sutton, et al. "Phytochemical and Genetic Analyses of Ancient Cannabis from Central Asia." *Journal of Experimental Botany* 59, no. 15 (November 2008): 4171–82. https://www.ncbi.nlm.nih.gov/pmc/articles/PMC2639026/.

Sagan, Carl. *The Dragons of Eden, Speculations on the Origin of Human Intelligence*. New York: Penguin Books, 1977.

Samuels, David. "Dr. Kush." *The New Yorker*, July 28, 2008. http://www.questia.com/read/1P3-1520182561/dr-kush.

Sayegh, Chris. "The Herbal Chef on Terpenes: Chris Sayegh Breaks Down These Fragrant, Flavorful Oils." *Dope*, July 30, 2017. http://www.dopemagazine.com/herbal-chef-terpenes-chris-sayegh-breaks-fragrant-flavorful-oils/.

Schack, T. Alan. "Report from Amsterdam: The New Breed of Coffeeshops." *High Times*, November 1994, 11.

Schultes, Richard Evans, and Albert Hofmann. *Plants of the Gods: Their Sacred, Healing and Hallucinogenic Powers.* New York: McGraw-Hill, 1979.

Schultes, Richard Evans, William M. Klein, Timothy Plowman, and Tom E. Lockwood. "Cannabis: An Example of Taxonomic Neglect." *Botanical Museum Leaflets, Harvard University* 23, no. 9 (February 28, 1974).

Sederberg, Christian. "Stories of Amendment 64 Oral History Project." Christian Sederberg, interviewed by Janet Bishop (Colorado State Library). https://dspace.library.colostate.edu/bitstream/handle/10217/176469/AMNT_OralHistoryTranscript_Sederberg-part2-sect2.pdf?sequence=11&isAllowed=y.

Sell, Charles S. *A Fragrant Introduction to Terpenoid Chemistry*. Ashford, Kent, UK: Quest International, 2003.

Small, Ernest, and Arthur Cronquist. "A Practical and Natural Taxonomy for Cannabis." *Taxon* 25, no. 4 (August 1976).

Small, Ernest, and David Marcus. "Hemp: A New Crop with New Uses for North America." In *Trends in New Crops and New Uses.* Alexandria, VA: ASHS Press, 2002.

Sokol, Zach. "A Stoned Swan Song: Scenes from the Lost Prohibition-Era Cannabis Competition in California, Where Big Weed Is Rising and Growers Are Getting Burnt." *Playboy*, 41–48.

Staggs, Brooke. "High Marijuana Taxes Spark Sticker Shock for California Cannabis Customers." *Pasadena Star-News*, January 26, 2018. http://www.questia.com/read/1P4-1991581406/high-marijuana-taxes-spark-sticker-shock-for-california.

Steinmetz, Katy. "420 Day: Why There Are So Many Different Names for Weed." *Time*, April 20, 2017. http://time.com/4747501/420-day-weed-marijuana-pot-slang/.

Steves, Rick. "Want to Smoke Marijuana in Spain? Join a Club." *Huffington Post*, May 24, 2016. https://www.huffingtonpost.com/rick-steves/want-to-smoke-marijuana-i_b_10121928.html.

Sula, Mike. "Herbal Notes Is Planting the Seeds of Culinary Cannabis in Chicago." *Chicago Reader*. https://www.chicagoreader.com/chicago/herbal-notes-culinary-cannabis-weed-dinners-manny-mendoza/Content?oid=45808759.

Sumner, William. "The Rise of Cannawine—Cannabis-Infused Wine." *Green Market Report*, April 4, 2018. https://www.greenmarketreport.com/the-rise-of-cannawine-cannabis-infused-wine/.

Taylor, Bayard. *The Lands of the Saracen.* New York: G. P. Putnam, 1863.

Toklas, Alice B. *The Alice B. Toklas Cook Book.* New York: Harper Perennial, 1954.

"Tony Bourdain—HAPPY PIZZA!!!!" YouTube video, 1:26, posted by Desiree West, March 8, 2011. https://www.youtube.com/watch?time_continue=81&v=8t2kvMIi8h0

Touw, Mia. "The Religious and Medicinal Uses of *Cannabis* in China, India and Tibet." *Journal of Psychoactive Drugs* 13, no. 1 (January–March 1981). https://www.cnsproductions.com/pdf/Touw.pdf.

Tovar, Juan Camilo Maldonado. "Meet the 'Father of Cannabis,' the Man Who Discovered Why Weed Makes You High." Vice.com, February 19, 2016. https://www.vice.com/en_us/article/mvxde4/raphael-mechulam-father-cannabis-discover-thc.

Tower, Jeremiah. *California Dish: What I Saw (and Cooked) at the American Culinary Revolution.* New York: Free Press, 2004.

Tvert, Mason. "Stories of Amendment 64 Oral History Project." Mason Tvert, interviewed by Janet Bishop (Colorado State Library). https://dspace.library.colostate.edu/bitstream/handle/10217/176472/AMNT_OralHistoryTranscript_Tverk-part3.pdf?sequence=3&isAllowed=y.

"Use of Marijuana Spreading in West, Poisonous Weed Is Being Sold Quite Freely in Pool Halls and Beer Gardens. Children Said to Buy It, Narcotic Bureau Officials Say Law Gives No Authority to Stop Traffic." *New York Times*, September 16, 1934, 6.

Valleriani, Jenna. "On Dutch Coffeeshops and Vancouver Dispensaries." *Lift*, January 13, 2016. https://news.lift.co/dutch-coffeeshops-canada-dispensaries/.

Vaughan, Roger. "Mad New Scene on Sunset, Strip." *Life*, August 26, 1966, 75–79.

"Vermonters Visit to Colorado to Study Legalized Marijuana." https://legislature.vermont.gov/assets/Documents/2016/WorkGroups/House%20Judiciary/Reports%20and%20Resources/W~Department%20of%20Public%20Safety~Vermonters%20Visit%20to%20Colorado%20to%20Study%20Legalized%20Marijuana~3-11-2015.pdf.

Victor, Daniel. "High Times Is Sold to Group That Includes Son of Bob Marley." *New York Times*, June 1, 2017. https://www.nytimes.com/2017/06/01/business/media/high-times-magazine-marijuana.html.

Viera, Lauren. "Better Than Pot Brownies, by a James Beard Award–Winning Chef." *New York Times Style Magazine*, March 24, 2016. https://www.nytimes.com/2016/03/24/t-magazine/marijuana-chocolate-candy-mindy-segal.html.

Vinkenoog, Simon. "Dutch Beat." *High Times*, June 1986, 53.

"Waiting to Inhale: Customers Pack Marijuana Store Reopening after U.S. Raid." *St. Louis Post-Dispatch (MO)*, January 16, 1997. http://www.questia.com/read/1P2-33047729/waiting-to-inhale-customers-pack-marijuana-store-reopening.

Wakefield, Dan. "The Prodigal Powers of Pot: Acclaimed by Ancients, Frowned on by Fuzz, Beatified by Beats, Marijuana Remains the Most Misunderstood Drug of All Time." *Playboy*, August 1962, 52–56.

Wallace, Alicia. "How One of America's Most Visible Fortune 1000 Giants Quietly Snuck into the Cannabis Industry." *The Cannabist*, September 22, 2016. HTTPS://WWW.THECANNABIST.CO/2016/09/22/SCOTTS-MIRACLE-GRO-CANNABIS-HAWTHORNE-GARDENING-CO-HYDROPONICS/61763/.

Wallace, Alicia. "Scotts Miracle-Gro in Talks with EPA about Marijuana Pesticides." *The Cannabist*, November 4, 2016. https://www.thecannabist.co/2016/11/04/scotts-marijuana-pesticides-epa-talks/66773/.

Wallace, Alicia. "Colorado Marijuana Sales Hit $1.5 Billion in 2017." *The Cannabist*, February 9, 2018. https://www.thecannabist.co/2018/02/09/colorado-rijuana-sales-december-year-2017/98606/.

Walsh, John, and Geoff Ramsey. "Uruguay's Drug Policy: Major Innovations, Major Challenges." Foreign Policy at Brookings, 2016. https://www.brookings.edu/wp-content/uploads/2016/07/Walsh-Uruguay-final.pdf.

Warf, Barney. "High Points: An Historical Geography of Cannabis." *Geographical Review* 104, no. 4 (2014).

Weed, Julie. "Move Over California—Canada's Opening Its Own $5B Cannabis Market in 2018." *Forbes*, December 18, 2017. https://www.forbes.com/sites/julieweed/2017/12/18/never-mind-california-canadas-opening-its-own-5b-cannabis-market-in-2018/#5e15f38a5ae6.

West, David P. "Hemp and Marijuana: Myths & Realities." North American Industrial Hemp Council, 1998. https://www.votehemp.com/PDF/myths_facts.pdf 3.

Whitfield, Chandra Thomas. "Capitalizing on Cannabis: Meet Colorado's Black 'Potrepreneurs.'" NBCNews.com, April 19, 2015. https://www.nbcnews.com/news/nbcblk/capitalizing-cannabis-meet-colorado-s-black-potrepreneurs-n344556.

Williams, Sean. "The Largest Pot Stock in the World Is Moving to the NYSE." May 21, 2018. https://www.fool.com/investing/2018/05/21/the-largest-pot-stock-in-the-world-is-moving-to-th.aspx.

Wilson, Scott. "Outlaw Weed Comes into the Light." *Washington Post*, March 16, 2018. https://www.washingtonpost.com/news/national/wp/2018/03/16/feature/californias-outlaw-marijuana-culture-faces-a-harsh-reckoning-legal-weed/?utm_term=.2d18a996b78b.

Winkler, Max. "Phnom Penh's Happy Pizza Left Me High and Dry." *Vice*, September 29, 2017. https://munchies.vice.com/en_us/article/mgxywp/phnom-penhs-happy-pizza-left-me-high-and-dry.

Wren, Christopher S. "Votes on Marijuana Are Stirring Debate." *New York Times*, November 17, 1996. https://www.nytimes.com/1996/11/17/us/votes-on-marijuana-are-stirring-debate.html.

Wright, Andy. "Beyond Brownies: The Science of Cooking with Cannabis." *The Splendid Table*, May 4, 2017. https://www.splendidtable.org/story/beyond-brownies-the-science-of-cooking-with-cannabis.

Xochi, Stoney. "Reflections from Barcelona: Spannabis 2017." *Cannabis Now*, March 28, 2017. https://cannabisnow.com/reflections-barcelona-spannabis-2017/.

Index

About the Author

Natural health and lifestyle expert **Robyn Griggs Lawrence** helped introduce mainstream America to sustainable, healthy lifestyles as editor-in-chief of *Natural Home* magazine for 11 years and introduced Western readers to the Japanese art of finding beauty in imperfection in her books *The Wabi-Sabi House* and *Simply Imperfect: Revisiting the Wabi-Sabi House.* She coauthored *7 Steps to a Safe, Nurturing Nursery* with Dr. Frank Lipman, MD.

She is now educating people about how to safely prepare and imbibe organic, sustainably grown cannabis for health and well-being. She wrote *The Cannabis Kitchen Cookbook*; is a contributing editor for *Sensi* magazine; and taught a popular course, "The Fundamentals of Cooking with Cannabis," for Green Flower Media. She teaches about the art of making cannabis food through workshops and catered events and shares recipes and other cannabis-related information as cannabis kitchen on Instagram.

Robyn was an editor with *Mother Earth News, Mountain Living, The Herb Companion,* and *Organic Spa* and ran successful blogs on *Huffington Post,* Care2.com, and Motherearthnews.com. A board member for the Center for Maximum Potential Building Systems in Austin, Texas, and an advisory board member for the Healthy House Institute, she's been featured in major media including the *New York Times, Bloomberg, Time, USA Today, Fast Company, The Guardian,* CNN, and others.

A certified yoga instructor focusing on yoga therapy for trauma and addiction, Lawrence is the mother of two incredible young adults. After living in Boulder, Colorado, for 25 years, she is currently a digital nomad, exploring and working in her Airstream.